KU-264-276

How to Save money on your horse's vet bills

By 'VET ON CALL'
RUSSELL LYON BVM&S, MRCVS

KENILWORTH PRESS

First published in Great Britain 2001 by
Kenilworth Press Ltd
Addington
Buckingham
MK18 2JR

075004

© R. Russell Lyon 2001

All rights reserved. No part of this publication may be reproduced,
stored in a retrieval system, or transmitted in any form or by any
means, electronic, mechanical, photocopying, recording or otherwise, without the prior permission of the copyright holder.

Cartoons from the collection of **FurSure® Enterprises,** Inc. USA,
Copyright FurSure® Enterprises, Inc. All Rights Reserved.

Illustrations on pages 77–79 by **Carole Vincer**

British Library Cataloguing in Publication Data
A CIP record for this book is available from the British Library

ISBN 1-872119-37-9

Typesetting and layout by Kenilworth Press
Printed and bound in Great Britain by Halstan and Co. Ltd

NORFOLK COLLEGE LIBRARY

3 8079 00075 094 3

THE AUTHOR

R
p
S
V
a
C
p
tl
w
le
h

THE COLLEGE of West Anglia

Landbeach Road • Milton • Cambridge

Tel: (01223) 860701

LEARNING *Centre*

The card holder is responsible for the return of this book

Fines will be charged on ALL late items

THE COLLEGE OF WEST ANGLIA

LEARNING CENTRE

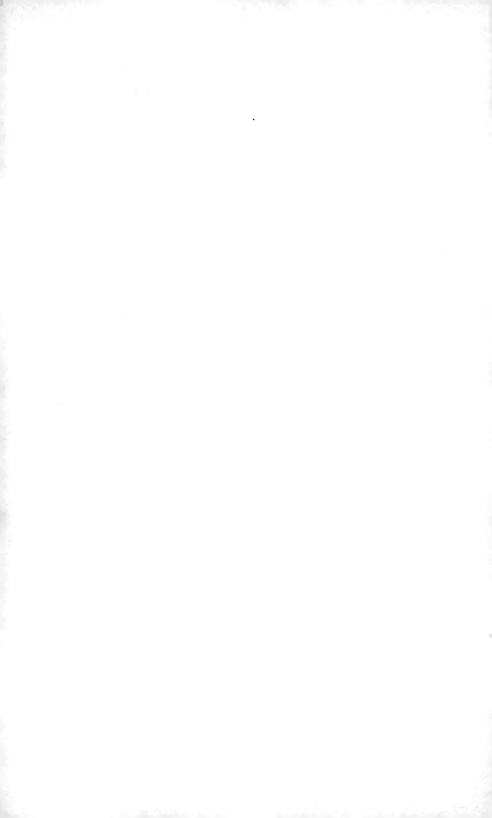

Contents

For Chris, with my love and thanks for her tolerance of my other 'woman' – my lap-top computer.

CHAPTER ONE

Know Your Horse, Your Vet – and Your Insurance Company

How well do you know your horse?

If you really want to save money on your horse's veterinary bills, the first thing to learn is the art of **observation**. Some people have an almost inbred ability to know and understand the animals they care for. Most of us, however, do not, but it is a skill that can be learned. Time spent leaning over a gate or a stable door and just admiring your horse is not time mis-spent if you are watching and learning.

If you know what is normal behaviour for your horse then you will instantly know what is not. That knowledge can save you money!

At its most basic, when you are mucking out in the morning you should be aware of whether the normal amount of droppings is present. If not, and you suspect that the animal may be becoming constipated, you can take swift and early action to remedy the situation. If you are being non-observant and action is not taken, you might fairly soon have a horse with impacted colic, which may require at best several expensive visits from the vet. Yet with care and observation many situations like this can be avoided, which is better for your animal and your bank balance.

If, like most people, you would like to become more aware of the habits and needs of your horse you must

> Learn to become so systematic with your observations that it becomes second nature to you.

learn to become so systematic with your observations that it becomes second nature to you. Start at the head end and make a point of noting every little detail you think is abnormal. Make notes if necessary. For example, a client quite recently noticed her horse had an eye discharge. She phoned and on my advice bathed the eye with dilute salt water for a few days. When it did not get better she again phoned and I recommended a visit. She had been very vigilant, and it was just as well – the animal had a tumour in its third eyelid. If the eye discharge had been ignored then the horse may well have lost its eye, or worse. As it was, all that was required was a fairly simple operation to remove the third eyelid, and the animal made a good recovery. The owner's diligence and good sense saved her horse a very serious operation, which would have been very expensive and may not have been totally successful.

A **thermometer** is a very useful piece of equipment. If you buy one from your veterinary practice, they will be very happy to teach you how to use it. You next have to get your horse used to the idea that just occasionally you'll want to insert something up its bottom. Most, as you might imagine, don't like the idea very much to begin with, but they will get used to the procedure quite quickly especially if it is accompanied by a bit of bribery in the form of a small amount of feed or a carrot. Knowing whether your animal has a temperature or not can be very useful in deciding whether to call the vet. A cough would, for

> Vets are almost always quite happy to dispense advice over the telephone, and such advice is still at the moment free.

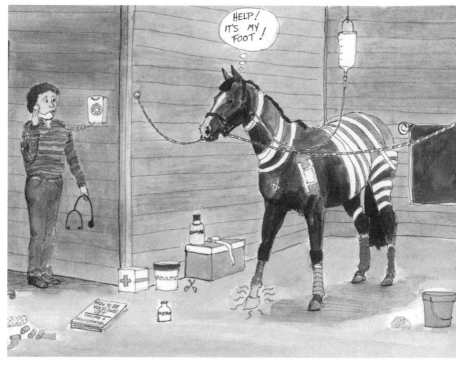

'Is that the vet? I think he wants to talk to you...'

example, be more to worry about if the animal was febrile (feverish) as well.

When a horse is very lame it is easy even for the novice to be able to spot which is the lame leg. When it is only slightly lame it becomes much more difficult. A self-evident fact about lameness is that the animal puts the lame leg to the ground for a shorter period of time than the other sound limbs. It becomes much easier to spot this if you get – as the vet does – someone to trot the animal up and down on a hard, level surface. It can also be useful to note that **the animal will lift its head up when a lame foreleg is on the ground; the head will go down when a lame hind leg is on the ground.** No one expects or wants owners to take the place of the vet but it can be handy to have an idea as to which leg is painful and to be able to give a good history of how long the lameness has been apparent when talking on the phone.

This sort of information is very helpful to a clinician when discussing a worry that a client might have. Vets are almost always quite happy to dispense advice over the telephone, and such advice is still at the moment free (unlike many solicitors!).

How well do you know your vet?

It is sensible to get to know your vet and build a good relationship with the veterinary practice you want to use. Don't chop and change practices unless you have very good reason. In this way it will be easier to arrange routine work such as vaccinations and tooth rasping that can be done at the same time. Even better, if you have a horse or horses at livery and know that other people in the yard use the same vet, **try to arrange a joint visit**, which can mean the call-out charge could be shared. Don't, however, wait until the vet calls to the yard to surprise him or her with these arrangements. Every vet I know hates to be greeted with 'while you are here can you just...?' It can mess up a morning round and is not popular, as it will make the vet late for the rest of the day, and even worse: – late for lunch! However, if it is arranged in advance, the vet will be happy, everyone will benefit and so will your pocket.

Taking your horse to the surgery is a great idea if your veterinary practice has facilities such as loose boxes at their premises – most equine practices do. When it comes to routine procedures such as lameness work-ups and X-rays, the vet will have all the facilities to hand and it will save professional time and you money, as there will be no call-out fee to pay. Don't always insist on a visit. It may be more appropriate and certainly cheaper to take the patient to the surgery.

Never forget that the vet is in business and needs to make a reasonable profit to survive. Practices are expensive to operate. Modern equipment is very costly; staff salaries are high, not to mention the overdraft. It is the vet's time that costs you, the client, money. The more time he or she spends on your yard (apart from drinking coffee) the more it will cost. **Have your animal caught, ready to be looked at and well presented.** Nothing makes a busy vet's heart sink more than to be met with, 'It's in the field – it won't take a minute to catch it,' when he or she knows darn well it will add at least another ten or fifteen minutes, at best, to the time of the visit – time which could be added on to your account.

While many horses in paddocks can be easily caught by their owners very many cannot, especially when it is the wrong time of day for coming in or when the more astute of them recognise – as many can – the vet. There is little more frustrating for the vet than wasting valuable time watching from a discreet distance while an owner or groom vainly tries to entice a reluctant or skittish animal into a headcollar. I have had to abort visits on quite a few occasions over the years, because the patient could not be caught. It was time wasted that had to be paid for, and the client had to pay a bill for a call-out which accomplished nothing. Take care that you do not get caught in the same way.

Ensure that you are insured

Every animal should be insured at the very least for **third-party damage.** Some years ago a client who had been on holiday came back to find that someone had left a gate open and two of his horses had strayed onto a busy road. The result was a disaster. One horse was killed and the other badly injured. Bad as that was it was not the main problem. The car involved was a write-off, and the driver injured and in hospital. The owner of the horse thought his horses were not insured for third-party risks and was very concerned that not only was he facing a large vet bill for his animals, but also that he was liable for the damage to the car and the driver. He didn't know whether he was covered for third-party risks as he had not specifically taken out such a policy. Luckily for him, when he checked he found that the health insurance he had on some of his animals meant they were all covered for third-party damage. This type of insurance is cheap, especially when it is tacked on to health insurance, and the consequences of not being covered could be ruinous. You may not be as lucky as my client. Don't leave it all to chance – check and be sure before an accident happens.

Health and life insurance for your horse can be expensive and you alone can make a judgment as to whether you wish to take out such policies. Treatment for your animal can be very expensive for, say, colic surgery. This can easily be at least £3,000 with no guarantee of success. The decision on whether to opt for surgery or not is so much easier if you know the horse is insured.

When deciding on a policy or a company it does not always make sense to go for the cheapest option. Many horse owners pay into health insurance for their animals for years only to find that they may not be covered when their need is greatest. If you are not sure which insurance company to use ask your vets which compa-

> **When deciding on a policy or a company it does not always make sense to go for the cheapest option.**

nies they would rather deal with. Many insurance companies have a long and honourable record of dealing with claims, but with some others it can be like getting a smile out of a traffic warden. **Don't be caught with the wrong policy or insurance company.**

Could you qualify for a discount?

Before you consent to an operation or diagnostic procedure for your horse, if you are worried about the possible costs involved, **ask for a quote or an estimate**. Be aware of the difference between the two. A written quote will give you exactly the amount of money you will have to pay. An estimate is different because it is not a hard-and-fast figure and could go up or down, depending on variable factors. If you believe your animal is insured for an operation, if it is not an emergency, check with the insurance company first before giving the go-ahead for surgery.

When you do get a bill please try to pay before the remittance becomes overdue. **You may even get a discount if you pay on time**; don't be afraid to ask, but don't overdo the haggling. Vets as a profession hate dealing with money and it is a major turn-off from the vet's point of view if he or she knows each visit is going to end with a row over money. If you have any problems with paying a bill, don't try to hide from it. Ring the practice and explain your difficulties, and in most cases you will be met with understanding; many will allow payment by instalments.

Keeping an animal is an expensive business but there are lots of ways to reduce the costs of veterinary treatment, which will not only have positive benefits for the health of your animal but also for your bank balance. **Prevention is always cheaper and better than cure**, as I will demonstrate in the forthcoming chapters.

CHAPTER TWO

Vaccination ... A Vet's Excuse to Make Money?

Vital statistics

There are thought to be over 600,000 horses and ponies in the United Kingdom. This is probably more than were in existence before the time of the internal combustion engine, although there are no statistics to prove the statement. It is fairly certain that equine numbers will continue to rise, given that the population as a whole is better off financially and has more spare time away from earning a living than ever before. Of these 600,000 animals less than thirty per cent receive any sort of vaccination at all, as most owners either think they can't afford it or don't believe it necessary. This means that in the UK at this moment **there are at least 420,000 animals without any protection against the most common equine diseases** such as tetanus, equine flu and equine herpes infection.

What is a vaccine?

Vaccines have advanced the fight of medicine against disease caused by bacteria and viruses. The earliest vaccines, such as were used against smallpox, were very crude but surprisingly effective. The smallpox vaccine was derived from cowpox lesions when it was realised that people who had been infected by this mild disease were protected from smallpox, which was a killer of millions.

The modern definition of a vaccine is that it is an

antigenic preparation used to stimulate the production of antibodies, which protect against one or more diseases. In lay terms this means that when an animal or human is vaccinated it is given a very mild form of the disease to stimulate the immune system in order to protect it from the real thing.

The evils of tetanus

Tetanus is a disease which has been around as long as there have been horses. It is still the most serious disease from which an animal can suffer and the horse is particularly susceptible to infection. It is caused by a bacterium, which is present in the soil – *Clostridium tetani* – and is especially abundant where horses are grazing.

I tend to see tetanus disease every two to three years and every time I encounter it I feel the same emotions as I did with my first case. I can see her now. She was a two-year-old part-bred Arab filly called Jenny. She was chestnut with a small star in the centre of her forehead, four white socks, and she was beautiful. She was also unvaccinated.

I was called to see her in the afternoon and found no external signs of injury, but she did, even to my then inexperienced eye, have early signs of tetanus. She was frightened, running a bit of a temperature and was beginning to dribble from the mouth as if swallowing was becoming a problem. Her nostrils were dilated, ears were erect and

> Many believe that if an animal is injected with antitoxin as soon as an injury or cut is discovered, then all will be well. This is very wrong. Over the years, of all the horses and ponies I have seen and treated for tetanus, I cannot recall ANY with external signs of injury.

> **Protecting your animals against tetanus is the most important thing you can do for them after feeding them, protecting them from inclement weather and foot care.**

when I tapped her forehead with my finger her third eyelids shot across her eyes faster than a ferret up a vet's trousers.

I gave her massive intravenous doses of penicillin, anti-tetanus serum and sedative. This was the standard treatment for tetanus, which has changed very little over the years, and I remember leaving her with no sense other than of acute foreboding for her welfare. A return visit a few hours later confirmed all my worst fears. She was dying, with all the horrors of the disease. She was on her side but partially propped up against a bale of straw, which was knocked away every time she had a convulsion. Unable to swallow due to the 'lock jaw' she looked, and I'm sure was, terrified. I put her out of her misery as soon as I could get the gun from the car.

Jenny's owner was devastated. He was not hard up for cash but he believed, like many others even today, that there is no need for routine vaccination against tetanus. He was aware of the disease but believed that if an animal is injected with antitoxin as soon as an injury or cut is discovered then all will be well. This is very wrong. Over the years, of all the horses and ponies I have seen and treated for tetanus, I cannot recall **any** with external signs of injury. It takes only a scratch, perhaps a thorn penetrating the skin, or a cut in the gum, for the tetanus bacillus to enter the tissues and for the poison to spread through the body. Tetanus germs are all around – in the soil – and are particularly prevalent where horses and ponies are grazing, as even healthy animals can be passing thousands of tetanus spores in their dung, which then contaminates the pasture.

Prevention of the disease is simple, straightforward and inexpensive. If you can't afford the vet's call-out fee, take the animal to the surgery or arrange a joint visit with a few like-minded friends who can share the visit cost. The vaccine is given by intramuscular injection, usually into the neck but another site such as into the brisket or hindquarters may be preferred. Two injections are given about six weeks apart. A booster jab is given a year later and then every two to three years thereafter. Most practices will send out reminders when a booster is due. If a mare is in foal she should be given a booster jab about four to six weeks before she is due to foal. In this way both she and the foal will be protected. If the mare is not vaccinated she should be given immediate protection within hours of giving birth by injecting her with tetanus antiserum. This is vital as the mare is very vulnerable after foaling – I know this too well, having experienced a mare dying from tetanus ten days after producing a healthy foal. The infection must have gained entry through the open birth canal. Foals born to mares that have not been properly protected or who may not have had adequate supplies of colostrum (the first milk that the mother produces and which is especially rich in antibodies) will also require injecting with antiserum within hours of birth. Foals born to mares that have been vaccinated at the correct times should not be vaccinated themselves until they are four to five months old.

Protecting your animals against tetanus is the most important thing you can do for them after feeding them, protecting them from inclement weather and foot care. Be sure you are not caught out. Check your vaccine certificate as soon as

> If you cannot afford to have your horse vaccinated against tetanus you really should not have bought it in the first place.

THE COLLEGE OF WEST ANGLIA

Learning Centre

possible and, if in doubt, double check with your vet. I have seen many animals die from tetanus. I have managed to save only two in all that time (thirty-plus years). Most die in terrified agony or have to be put down when they become recumbent and cannot swallow or breathe as the toxin paralyses their muscles. If you cannot afford to have your horse vaccinated against tetanus you really should not have bought it in the first place. **This form of vaccination is cheap and should never be neglected.** It is not a vet's perk. Get it done!

Equine flu – weighing up the risks

A few months ago I was invited to the launch of an updated version of an equine flu vaccine. There was a series of presentations pertinent to the occasion given by four experts. These gave me much to think about and I gained a new insight into the work which goes on behind the scenes before a new product arrives in the veterinary practice. It also made me stop and think on the advice I have been giving clients over the years.

Equine flu at its worst is a highly infectious disease, which causes high temperatures, aching muscles and a severe, dry cough which can last for two or more weeks. Most infected animals show very little inclination to eat and appear very depressed. In short, it is very like the human version of flu, and if you have ever been a sufferer of a flu infection you will know only too well how a horse or pony will feel – miserable. And *you* know what the problem is, *they* don't!

Young animals are usually the most severely affected and the most likely to develop side-effects, but older horses, like old people, can also be very vulnerable. The vast majority of patients make a good recovery but complications such as pneumonia or pleurisy and even

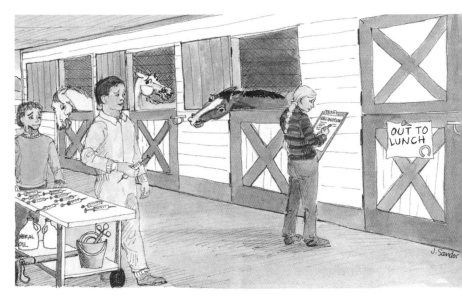

The annual vaccination round.

damage to the heart can occur, especially if precautions to minimise the effects of the disease are not taken.

The first flu outbreak I witnessed and was called upon to treat happened in the late 1970s. There were about sixty horses in the yard – all show jumpers – and the infection went around nearly all the animals in less than three days. This is not surprising really when you know that when a horse coughs, infectious particles can carry (without any wind assistance) at least thirty metres. The few that escaped illness had been vaccinated, but others who had been injected succumbed to the virus. The source of the infection seemed to be some German horses, which had been imported especially for an international competition.

I found that injecting antibiotics into patients made very little difference to the course of the disease, which was to be expected as antibiotics have no effect on viruses and are only useful in countering secondary bacterial infections that cause pneumonia. The most important contribution I made to the animals' welfare was to try and ensure that all the patients had plenty of fresh air and rest. Dusty boxes were avoided if at all possible. Hay was soaked for thirty minutes before being drained and fed. All patients were confined in loose boxes and only walked a short distance twice a day.

Now there are drugs available, which can help to alleviate the worst symptoms of respiratory distress. Drugs such as Ventipulmin and Sputulosim were not at that time available, but I'm sure fresh air and good nursing care were as vital to the horse's recovery then as they are now. After a bout of flu, once the animal has recovered from the acute symptoms it will often be under par for some time, and it can be disastrous for the horse's general health if it is returned to work too soon. An early return to work can lead to poor performances, and in highly competitive fields such as racing this can be very serious. It is not surprising that the horse racing world takes equine flu very seriously and vaccination is mandatory on all racing yards.

I suspect that many horse owners have their animals vaccinated solely in order not to be excluded from major sporting events. How many have experienced the embarrassment of being turned away at the showground gate for failing to have correct flu vaccination documents? Many then phone their veterinary practice in high dudgeon, as the vet is often blamed for inadequate or incorrect certificates. While this sometimes may be the case it is up to the individual owner to be sure before he or she embarks on a long journey or sends in entry forms that vaccinations are up to date and correct.

> **Equine flu – it can be disastrous for the horse's general health if it is returned to work too soon.**

Flu vaccine is usually given from the age of five months in two injections six weeks apart. A booster is then injected six months later and then given annually. This is usually combined with tetanus protection. The yearly booster must not be late, and must be given not more than a year after the previous injection. If this is not the case, the certificate will be invalid and the animal may be refused entry to an event. **If your certificate is out of date you will be obliged to start the injection procedure all over again, which is a costly mistake to make.** Some veterinary practices send out reminders at the correct time – but do not rely on this as mistakes can happen and post may be delayed. It is not the vet's job to remind you to keep your horse's jabs up to date – that is the owner's (or the groom's) responsibility.

When the animal is vaccinated for the first time make sure that the vet fills in the description on the document. It is common for a busy vet to say he or she will do it the next time, but when the next time comes a different vet arrives and he/she cannot certify what another has done. You then have to go back to the first vet to get the document completed. This is a waste of time and may, although it should not, cost you extra money.

If your certificate is out of date don't be tempted to ask the vet to back-date the document. It will offend the vet you ask and any such request will be refused, as it would constitute a fraud. The Royal College of Veterinary Surgeons takes – quite rightly – a very dim view of any professional person issuing a document knowing it to be fraudulent.

Horse owners often ask me if there is any point in having their animals vaccinated against flu, as 'they never go anywhere'. This is easily countered, as even if the animal doesn't go to external events it will almost certainly meet others who do. Another common excuse for not vaccinating is age. Many believe that to flu vaccinate an old horse is a waste of money. If this were the case with humans, then the NHS could save a lot of cash, as it tends to reserve the use of vaccine for the old and vulnerable.

In the past I tended to think that the equine flu virus had altered little over the years, but this does not appear to be the case. There are several different strains of the virus, and vaccine companies spend a lot of time and money keeping up with the various forms, which seem to appear with yearly regularity. For example, virus strains of American lineage are now appearing again with greater frequency in Europe. In fact, in the last two years, the majority of outbreaks in Europe have been identified as American type, and some of the older types of vaccine will not completely protect your horse. Your vet should be in the best position to know whether the vaccine your animal is about to receive is fully up to date. If he or she is not sure, it is straightforward for a vet to find out by phoning the vaccine companies for current information on their products.

Another point which came out at the vaccine meeting I attended was that it might be better to delay vaccinating youngsters against flu until they are nine months old. Current research has shown that at this age the vaccine – any flu vaccine – gives a much stronger immunity. This, however, does not mean that tetanus vaccination should be delayed. This must be done, as already explained, from four to five months of age if the mother has been properly vaccinated, and from three months if not. It still shocks me to know that less than thirty per cent of British horses are vaccinated against tetanus. Not to vaccinate against flu is more understandable, as it is relatively expensive and is a disease from which most animals recover, but not to vaccinate against tetanus in my opinion is almost tantamount to criminal neglect and without excuse at all.

Herpes virus infections

Herpes virus infections can cause a variety of symptoms depending on which strain of the virus is involved. At present there are four distinct strains of equine herpes virus (EHV), of which EHV1 is the most dangerous and virulent. There are two subtypes of this EHV1 strain. One causes abortion and the other causes respiratory symptoms.

It is this respiratory subtype and also the EHV4 strain, which the average horse owner is most likely to encounter. The symptoms are unremarkable. Three days from the initial infection there is a thin, watery discharge from the nose, which is usually accompanied by an occasional cough and a mild temperature. After about a week, the animal may get a secondary bacterial infection, the discharge from the nose may become purulent, the cough more persistent and pneumonia can be the result.

I attended an outbreak of this type of infection two years ago where the initial viral infection was complicated by strangles (see later), which attacked some debilitated patients and resulted in one death.

As a general rule most animals will make a complete, if slow, recovery. However, besides the risk of pneumonia in all the horses it affects, there is the ever–present threat that it can cause a mare to abort. There is also a much more rare but still significant risk of the paralytic form of the disease. Symptoms of this are a sudden loss of coordination and paralysis of the hind legs, and it all too often proves untreatable and fatal. If a horse is found cast in a box and is unable to stand, a blood test should

> Herpes virus vaccination? If you keep your horse with many others, such as in a large livery yard, then it could be money well spent.

be taken at the outset to preclude the possibility of an acute herpes infection.

Diagnosis of the respiratory form of the disease can be difficult, as it cannot be confirmed on clinical signs alone. In the very early stages of the infection, the virus can be recovered from swabs taken from the windpipe. By the time secondary bacterial infections are in place, this is not possible and the only way then to make a firm diagnosis is by serological tests on blood serum. This requires two blood samples. The first is taken at the outset of the disease and the second two to three weeks later. A four-fold increase in the levels of antibodies in the second sample is proof positive of infection by the herpes virus.

Treatment of the respiratory form of the disease has to be under the direction of the vet who will normally prescribe antibiotics as a precaution against secondary bacterial infection, as well as other medication which might be required to help breathing and get rid of excess phlegm and mucus from the airways. This can cost quite a lot of money, which if you are insured may not be too much of a problem, but routine vaccination against the EHV1 and EHV4, which has become available only comparatively recently, is very much cheaper. The vaccine has to be given, like flu and tetanus, as two injections six weeks apart and then as six-monthly boosters. The percentage uptake of this vaccine in the horse population is very low and while it may not be appropriate to vaccinate in every situation, if you keep your horse with many others, such as in a large livery yard, then I would suggest it could be money well spent.

Strangles

There are certain things you learn from life – and some quicker than others. These are the things that no one tells you about – you have to discover them for yourself; and when you do, you never forget. An example of this is how to lance an abscess. The 'how to do it' is taught in veterinary college. Other matters, such as standing a safe distance away with your mouth shut, are something you have to learn for yourself. I found this out the hard way when I had to lance a large fulminating abscess in a yearling's neck. I merely touched the skin with the scalpel when it erupted like an angry volcano and purulent material covered me from head to toe. It was in my face, mouth, my hair, and my eyes, and was most unpleasant.

The disease the animal was suffering from was strangles. It's a word that strikes fear into most horse owners. Possibly this is because of the emotive name, and also because, before penicillin was discovered, very many horses died of the disease.

Strangles is a bacterial disease caused by *Streptococcus equi,* which is specific to horses and ponies. Infection in the early stages results in a high temperature, a soft cough and a muco-purulent nasal discharge. As the disease progresses, the lymph nodes in the head and neck become swollen, making swallowing difficult, and it can also impair breathing.

The patient I have already mentioned was a youngster, a bay filly about sixteen months old. She was part of a group in a yard who one by one went down with the infection. The older animals were not too badly affected. Two did not have any symptoms, and a third required only one injection of penicillin to put it right.

The others, all up to six years old, had soft coughs and purulent nasal discharges. They all responded very well to a series of penicillin injections, with one exception. The filly developed, despite initial antibiotic treatment, large swellings in the neck just behind the jaw. I stopped antibiotic treatment for a day or two, which the owner thought a perverse thing to do, but I wanted the abscesses to come to a head so that they would either burst of their own volition or be lanced. The animal became very poorly with a high temperature and I visited it early one evening hoping the time had come to lance the abscesses. It was. If I had been an hour or two later, I'm sure they would have burst. As it was I lanced them with the results I have already described. My annoyance at myself for getting covered in pus was somewhat alleviated by an almost instant improvement in the filly's condition.

Within ten minutes her temperature had dropped to virtually normal, she wanted something to eat, and was most upset when I gave her another injection. I knew the antibiotic would work well this time as it would not be overwhelmed by purulent material and would mop up the rest of the bacteria.

Within a few days the patient was almost back to normal and every one was very relieved. However, I was concerned in case she or one of the others might develop a condition called 'bastard strangles'. This is where the infection causes abscesses to appear in the internal organs, such as the mesenteric lymph nodes of the gut, liver or spleen. This can be very serious even today and the animal has very little chance of making a full recovery.

Most horse owners are aware that the disease is very infectious. The bacteria can be shed from draining abscesses and nostrils for up to four weeks and can remain viable on tack, clothing or indeed any surface for many months. Ideally all animals in contact with a proven case should be isolated. I also tend to give all animals that have been in contact an injection of long-acting penicillin. This at the moment, apart from disinfecting everything in sight, is all that can be done to limit an outbreak of the disease.

When I first qualified there was a vaccine available against strangles but this was not very effective and was discontinued. However, I do understand that a new strangles vaccine may be about to come on the market. When it is produced commercially it may be worthwhile, in certain parts of the country, to vaccinate youngstock against the disease, as they are most at risk. If in doubt about the availability and necessity for vaccination, check with your veterinary surgeon.

If you are in the business of breeding horses, vaccines are available to prevent abortions caused by **equine arteritis** and to boost the immunity of foals to **rotavirus infection** that results in diarrhoea, but this is a specialised field and beyond the present remit of this book.

A bad reaction?

Vaccine reactions used to be quite commonplace. It was not unusual for a number of horses or ponies to have a sore neck after a vaccine jab. This is far less likely today as modern vaccines are not only far more effective but much less likely to cause a reaction. But it still can happen.

Many vets, myself included, will often vaccinate a patient into the pectoral muscles in front of the chest rather than into the neck. If a reaction happens then the horse is still able to eat. If you know your animal has had a sore neck in the past then remind the vet to give the vaccine elsewhere as a horse or pony with a sore neck has great difficulty in grazing, and food usually has to be fed from an elevated manger. Very occasionally, if I am feeling brave, I will put vaccine into the horse's backside. The only reaction I have ever experienced with this method is the kick that goes with the jab. If a horse is quite poorly after a vaccination, the vaccine company will sometimes, if asked nicely by your vet, help towards the cost of the treatment.

Severe allergic reactions to a vaccine are fortunately very rare indeed but can still occur. The worst I ever experienced within the practice happened about ten years ago. A colleague was called to vaccinate a group of Welsh mares, most of whom were pregnant.

Pregnant mares are vaccinated very frequently as it is a very safe procedure but all manufacturers have a let-out clause that states that while their vaccine is perfectly safe, handling pregnant mares carries its own inherent risk.

All the animals in the group had their injections without too much trouble. In fact, they were all so well behaved, they were done in the field. One mare, however, kicked up her heels after her injection and galloped off across the paddock. Nothing was thought out of the ordinary at the time but within the hour she was found, to everybody's distress, dead.

> If a horse is quite poorly after a vaccination, the vaccine company will sometimes help towards the cost of the treatment.

A comprehensive post-mortem was carried out and many samples were taken for laboratory examination. The vaccine makers were alerted that a horse had died very shortly after injection and instantly agreed to pay the full costs of the investigation. The tests proved that the cause of the death was an allergic or anaphylactic reaction to the vaccine and nothing to do with the pregnancy. It is possible had the mare been kept under observation for a few minutes and the symptoms observed, her life could have been saved by an intravenous injection of soluble corticosteroids or adrenaline given intramuscularly. It is for just this possibility that all humans are asked to sit quietly in the doctor's waiting room after being vaccinated, for fifteen minutes or so to make sure that if there is a reaction, help is at hand.

When the vaccine makers were aware of the findings, although it was no fault of the vaccine, they agreed 'as a gesture of good will' to compensate the owner for the dead mare and the dead foal. This sad incident should not deter you from using vaccine to protect your horses. The benefits conferred far outweigh any possible risks and I am still using the same company's vaccine to this day.

A word of advice

Be selective in your choice of vaccination – apart from tetanus. Ask your veterinary practice (they won't mind, I promise!) which vaccinations are most appropriate for your horses and your situation. That way you will get the best value for your money.

CHAPTER THREE

Are Wormers a Waste of Money?

Don't wriggle out of this one

Wormers are not a waste of money, they are essential for the health of your horse, but if you use the wrong wormer at the wrong time and at the wrong dose you might just as well chuck your money on the muck-heap!

Intestinal parasites (worms) have been present in horses and ponies as long as equines themselves have existed. These parasites vary enormously and often have very different life-cycles. They are often as diverse and different as a sheep is different from a dog. They tend to be classified according to their life-cycles and can be put into three groups:

- roundworms (nematodes)
- tapeworms (cestodes), and
- flukes (trematodes) – these parasites infect horses only very rarely but are common in sheep, and less so in cattle.

Most of us are aware that horses have worms and should be de-wormed on a regular basis. Some people use wormers twice a year, and others, with almost religious fervour, use an anthelmintic every six weeks, winter and summer, 'whether the horse needs it or not'. Many horse owners are also aware that they should not use the same product on their animals all the time, which often means they use a different preparation every six weeks, which can be quite the wrong thing to do. It is fortunate that today there is a wide range of very effective drugs, which can be used against internal parasites – but no one wormer is effective against all types of parasites.

> **If you use the wrong wormer at the wrong time and at the wrong dose you might just as well chuck your money on the muck-heap.**

What is certain is that no two situations are the same. What may be the correct worming regime for one horse owner may be totally wrong or inadequate for another only a few fields away. A horse grazing in a field of twenty acres with one other companion and a few sheep will be at much less risk than another which is in a six-acre paddock with many other horses for company.

Above all, horse owners need to think about what they are doing and work out a sensible treatment regime with their vet and not pick one or two wormers which a friend 'swears by' or which can be bought at a very good price. There are more misconceptions about wormers and worming than almost any other form of equine medicine. Unfortunately there are no statistics available to back my assertion but I know from personal experience in my practice, dealing with the problem all the time – summer and winter – that taken as a whole **many hundreds of British horses die every year from the effects of internal parasites.** These deaths could so easily and relatively cheaply be prevented. They either die from colic or debility as the result of wasting or acute diarrhoea. In many cases these are animals that have received anthelmintic treatment but not

> **There are more misconceptions about wormers and worming than almost any other form of equine medicine.**

A horse that has not been de-wormed could easily be passing over 10 MILLION parasite eggs per week.

the correct drug or correct dose or at the appropriate time. Please remember that no single wormer can control all the internal parasites in the horse. Wormers given without much thought and hoping for the best may well be a total waste of money.

One way of finding out whether your animal is heavily parasitised is to have a faecal **worm egg count** done on fresh droppings. This is a comparatively simple test, which will tell you how many parasite eggs per gram are being passed in the faeces. Your veterinary practice may have a laboratory which can carry out the test, but if not will send it on to an outside specialist. You may well be horrified by the result if you have this done in the summer months, as many thousands of worm eggs per gram of faeces are not uncommon. The mathematics can be terrifying. If a horse is passing even a small number of worm eggs, say, one hundred per gram, and the animal passes about 15kg of dung in a day, this means that **one and half million eggs are being passed daily** onto the pasture. If you add this up per week it could be that a horse that has not been de-wormed could easily be passing over ten million parasite eggs per week, each one a potential threat!

In the winter months when the weather is cold, the parasite life-cycle slows dramatically and immature worms become encysted and dormant in the wall of the intestine. Worm egg counts can diminish to almost zero but it is in the winter months that many internal parasites can cause the worst damage to the host animal.

A **blood sample** can be more helpful during these cold months to help determine the degree of parasitism in the animal and give a more accurate idea of a potential problem.

It is also possible to have the soil in the pasture or paddock analysed to check on the degree of parasitic pasture contamination. Your vet can arrange to have this done; also the Depart of Environment, Food and Rural Affairs specialist laboratories (ADAS) usually provide this type of service.

There is much a client can do to be alert to the signs of high worm burdens in their own horses and ponies. Initially the symptoms, whatever the season, are a loss of condition and weight, which can be sudden or gradual, a lack of appetite, and a general unthrifty look with a dull coat. The animal may become lethargic and have filled legs (also abdomen and sheath if a gelding or stallion). Foals that are heavily parasitised may also have a pot-belly as well as a staring coat. It is **always** too late to wait until the animal has a severe attack of colic or diarrhoea before taking action: the patient can so easily die.

Red worms

Red worms (nematodes) are the most common internal parasite of the horse. These worms can be further subdivided into **large red worms** (*Strongylus vulgaris* and *Strongylus edentatus*) and small red worms (**Cyathostomes**). Both types of red worm can cause severe disease and in the right circumstances are killers.

Two winters ago I attended a young Percheron stallion. He was in the early stages of colic. He was sweating a bit, had a raised pulse and an anxious expression. I had a listen to his gut sounds, which were a bit reduced but not serious, and he allowed me to examine him per rectum without becoming too distressed. The rectal examination indicated that he was neither consti-

> **Both types of red worm can cause severe disease and in the right circumstances are killers.**

pated nor had diarrhoea, which suggested he had a spasmodic colic. All this means is that he had intermittent pain in his abdomen, which was gut related. Most cases of spasmodic colic respond well to muscle relaxant and pain-killing drugs, but it is known that a very high percentage (at least eighty per cent) are due to red worm larvae migrating up the mesenteric artery of the intestine. This causes a total or partial obstruction of the blood supply to the bowel, which reacts by going into a spasm, and the animal can experience acute and agonising pain.

I went back to the car to get syringe, needle and some Buscopan, which I use frequently for such cases. By the time I got back – it was only a few minutes – the horse had got down, and despite the owner's best efforts to get him to his feet, had rolled twice.

The clinical picture changed dramatically in those few moments. The stallion had began to sweat profusely, the pulse rate rose dramatically and when I applied the stethoscope to his abdomen to have another listen to his gut movements, he kicked me instantly and very hard. (If a heavy horse weighing about a ton has never kicked you, I can tell you it is not to be recommended. If the kick had just been a few inches lower my thigh bone would have been snapped like a twig. As it was I nursed a massive bruise on my hip for weeks.) Only a few moments before, the animal had allowed a rectal examination but now the situation had become critical. After sedating him and relieving his agony at least a little, on further examination, it became clear that the spasm of the bowel had resulted in the intestines becoming twisted. The farmer was quite convinced this had happened because he had allowed the animal to roll but, more likely, the gut twisted first then the horse went down.

Whatever the sequence of events it had now become clear that the stallion either had to have emergency surgery or would have to be put down. The nearest equine operating theatre was about forty miles away and in addition I had to tell the owner that the likely cost of such an operation would probably be at least £2,000 to £3,000. This would have to be paid whether the animal survived or not, and I estimated the odds at the time to be no better than 50/50.

Unfortunately the horse was not insured and economics had to be taken into account. In the end I had to shoot the poor beast. I can tell you that putting a horse down is the worst job I have to do as a vet. I never fail to feel sick every time I put the gun to a forehead and pull the trigger. It was made all the worse in this instance by the fact, which I told the farmer later, was that his horse would not have had colic if he had wormed it properly and regularly with the correct wormer. The post-mortem had proved the cause of the colic to be migrating larvae in the mesenteric artery. This larva was only a few millimetres in size and yet it had managed to kill a magnificent horse weighing just under a ton. What made the case even more difficult was knowing that had it been dewormed properly with an Ivermectin drug such as Eqvalan, which doesn't cost any more than a couple of cinema tickets for a syringe, the animal would not have had colic in the first place. The farmer had wormed all his horses just two or three weeks before but with a type which has no effect on migrating larvae. He did not de-worm as routine but only when he thought his horses looked as if they needed

> **At least 80% of all cases of spasmodic colic are due to red worm larvae.**

to be wormed. It was an expensive and sad lesson for him, and one he would never forget.

Lethal though large red worms can be, they cause less trouble to the equine world than small red worms – the **Cyathostomes**. These worms are far more deadly because of their life-cycle. In the autumn after the larvae have been picked up from the pasture while the horse is grazing, the larvae in its third stage of development becomes encysted in the cells of the gut wall. While it is there it is effectively hiding and is very difficult to treat. If left untreated, come the late winter or early spring when conditions are right for the parasite, they resume their growth. The simultaneous emergence of possibly thousands of fourth stage larvae can cause devastating damage to the wall of the large intestine, which can in many cases result in the death of the horse.

The worst example of this I have ever seen was in two Thoroughbred yearlings. They were found in a field by an RSPCA inspector, along with a few other apparently healthy horses. The inspector was following up a complaint by a member of the public. This unfortunate pair of animals were skeletal. I have never seen two animals look so thin, and they were scouring so badly the diarrhoea was pouring out of them like water. Investigation proved that the animals were suffering from cyathostomiasis, and that they must have lost condition very rapidly. Despite intensive treatment, which cost many hundreds of pounds, one animal died within twenty-four hours and the other was destroyed two days later when it became clear that it was suffering badly and recovery was most unlikely.

> **Small red worms are more deadly than large red worms, because of their life-cycle.**

Every horse should be treated for Cyathostomes in the late autumn and again in late spring. This usually involves dosing with Panacur Guard for five days in late October or early November, to remove encysted larvae acquired during the summer, and again in February to remove those that have been picked up in the winter months or that have hidden successfully in the lining of the intestines. An Ivermectin drug called Equest can also be useful in this role but is only effective against the more mature third stages of the larvae. These wormers, which cost no more than the price of an Indian take-away for two, are very effective and must be worth the price of a horse.

More uninvited guests
Ascarids are large round worms and can reach as long as 30cm (1 ft) when mature and produce large numbers of tough-coated eggs. These eggs are microscopic in size but very infective to foals. The worm eggs, which can be found sticking to the coat and udder of the lactating mare, can become adult within about twelve weeks of infection and block or rupture a foal's small intestine, with sometimes deadly results. Part of the worm's life-cycle is to migrate through the lung and they can, due to this migration, cause severe coughing in a youngster. For this reason it is vital that new foals are treated for worms within six weeks of age. Most of the popular range of anti-worming drugs are effective against ascarids. By the time the animal is about two years old the youngster will have developed a solid immunity to the round worm.

Scouring in the new foal is often attributed to the hormonal changes that occur in the mare when she comes into season. While this may be a factor in some cases many causes of diarrhoea are due to infection of the foal by another round-worm parasite called *Strongyloides westeri*. This infection is passed to the foal from the mother through the milk and can result in severe scouring. Fortunately it is a parasite which is easily treated by dosing the foal, and prevented by de-worming the mare before she gives birth.

Lungworm (*Dictyocaulus arnfieldi*), another round worm, used to be a severe and intractable problem in horses when they were grazed with donkeys. For many years there were no drugs available which would kill the parasite, and although the worm does not seem to have any harmful effects on the donkey it can live in the air passages of the lungs of horses and ponies and cause a hard, hacking cough. Fortunately modern anthelmintics such as Eqvalan, Equest or Panacur are very effective against this parasite.

For a long time **tapeworm** (*Anoplocephala perfoliata*) in horses was not thought to be very significant. For years it was believed to be a fairly harmless parasite but recent evidence has tended to implicate the tapeworm in causing some types of colic. It has been said that up to 20 per cent of surgical colic cases have been the result of tapeworm infection causing inflammation and irritation at the ilio-caecal junction. The intermediate host of the worm is the forage mite, which survives on spring and summer pasture, and on hay and bedding during the winter months. The horse is thus exposed to infection all the year round so that worming control every six months is vital to

Just because you can't see any tapeworm segments does not mean your horse is not infected.

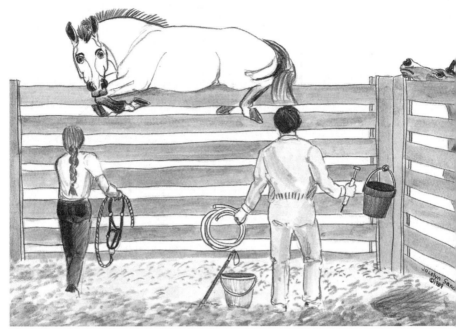

'No, really ... I feel fine now.'

control the parasite.

Most internal parasites cannot be seen by the naked eye when they are passed in the dung. However, tapeworm segments are one of the exceptions to this and are readily seen as small white, usually square or rectangular, particles on the surface of expelled dung. However, just because you can't see any segments does not mean your horse is not infected, and routine worming should always be carried out. Strongid P or Pyratape P given at double the normal dose are the only effective treatments for tapeworm, and should be given in the spring and autumn every year.

Pin worms or *Oxyuris equi* are very common but not thought to be a serious pathogen (disease-causing agent). The adult worms are found in the large intestine, and the females migrate to the anus where they lay large numbers of sticky eggs. These cause irritation and a severe itch so that the infected animal spends most of its time rubbing its backside on any available post or stable fitting. In the summer months it can be easy to confuse this irritation with sweet itch, but the itch is confined to the hindquarters only and most of the broad-spectrum anthelmintics will get rid of the parasite. Any horse with the eggs (clusters of eggs look like grey jelly) stuck around its bottom will get immediate relief by having them cleaned away with a disposable cloth.

Bots are not actually true worms; they are bot fly larvae and they live in the horse's stomach. They look like large maggots and are thought to live off the horse's food for about ten months of the year. The adult fly is active in early summer and September. It lays its eggs on the hairs of the horse or pony, which are then ingested by the animal when it grooms the body by licking. The larvae migrate through the animal's internal organs and then arrive in the stomach, where they can cause inflammation, digestive disorders and colic.

Fortunately any of the Ivermectin group of drugs (Eqvalan, Equest or Panomec) is effective in getting rid of the pest, but it is best to wait until December, by which time the frosts should have killed the bot flies and the bot larvae have reached the stomach.

In addition to those significant pathogens there are others such as
• the **stomach hairworm** (*Trichostrongylus axei*),
• the **large-mouthed stomach worm** (*Habronema muscae*), and
• the **neck threadworm** (*Onchocerca*),
which are common in horses, but not especially signifi-

cant, and all are readily treated, if necessary, by Eqvalan or Equest.

Your best defence

A **strategic worming programme** will need to be adaptable to suit individual requirements and should ideally be discussed with your vet. Your veterinary practice will be happy to discuss a worming programme with you, especially if you buy the drugs from the practice.

I find it best to divide a worming schedule into the summer and winter periods.

WORMING SCHEDULE

Summer

There are three chemically different wormers available for treating horses and ponies. These are

(1) the **Benzimidazole** group, such as Panacur, Telmin and Systamex (and many others);

(2) the **Ivermectin** group, which includes Eqvalan, Equest and Panomec; and

(3) **Pyrantel**, which is the active ingredient in Strongid P and Pyratape P.

Between April and August you should use **one of these chemically different wormers on an annual basis and as part of a three-year cycle.**

By rotating the anthelmintic drug every year, not every dose, you reduce the risk of resistance developing in the worms to the drug used.

Year 1: Use a Benzimidazole wormer (e.g. Panacur, Telmin, Systamex or similar) every four to six weeks.

Year 2: Use Strongid P or Pyratape P every four to six weeks.

Year 3: Use Panomec, Eqvalan or Equest. Panomec or Eqvalan can be used every eight to ten weeks, and if using Equest the manufacturers state that every thirteen weeks should be adequate.

Winter

As far as the winter worming programme is concerned this should commence in **September** with a double dose of Strongid P or Pyratape P as these are the only products effective against tapeworm.

In **October/November** use Panacur Guard or double the normal dose of the standard Panacur preparation for five consecutive days. This is still the only licensed product against the early stages of the encysted small red worm and will also be helpful in eliminating migrating large red worm larvae. Some authorities may advocate the use of Equest at this stage, and whilst it does have a role to play it is claimed to be effective only against the more mature larvae in the gut wall.

December is the time to use an Ivermectin product (Panomec, Eqvalan or Equest), as they are not only highly effective anthelmintics but they are also the only products that will effectively get rid of stomach bots.

In **mid-February** use Panacur Guard again to remove any small red worm larvae that may have been acquired during the winter months or that were missed by the November dose. This de-worming will also help reduce the level of worms on the pasture in the spring.

March means the double dose of Pyratape P or Strongid

P again for tapeworm before reverting in April to the summer regime.

This programme has been the basis of the advice tendered by my practice in the last two to three years but may have to be altered to suit individual situations. Your horses may have a known resistance to some of the drugs I have mentioned. The Benzimidazole group are especially at risk of this occurring, and if this is the case you will require advice from your vet as to how to alter the worming programme. If you are worried about drug resistance ask your vet to do a faecal egg count reduction test. Samples are taken on the day of worming and then again seven to twenty-one days later. If resistance is present, then that wormer should not be used during the grazing season, although it may still be required for specific strategic dosing, such as for Cyathostomes.

Don't be afraid to de-worm a pregnant mare. All the de-wormers mentioned are safe for use in pregnancy.

All horses and ponies using the same grazing should be de-wormed with the same product and at the same time. This is not always easy to arrange in a livery yard but is well worth the effort.

Get tough with worms!
While anthelmintic drugs are a necessary expense when you own a horse or pony, there is much that can be done to reduce the worm burden on your pasture and in your animal that doesn't cost you any money. It is unwise to rely totally on wormers to control parasites, as no drug treatment, no matter how good, is likely to be one hundred per cent effective. Effective pasture management is just as vital as using the best wormers and is very cost-efficient.

> Effective pasture management is just as vital as using the best wormers and is very cost-efficient.

The regular removal of dung from pasture is the single most effective means of reducing the worm burden on that paddock. This should be done twice a week in both summer and winter, as it is essential to keep the level of infective larvae as low as possible. It is very common to overstock horses in the winter months (the ideal in my opinion is one horse per acre), especially in turn-out paddocks, and it would be best if at all possible in this situation to collect the dung daily. If time is scarce, as it often is in short winter days, concentrate on removing dung from paddocks where the youngsters are turned out.

Mixed grazing, using cattle and sheep, can be very useful for reducing pasture contamination. Sheep and cattle eat the horse worms and vice versa and there is no cross-over with infection. They are also very effective at improving the quality of the grass, as they will eat much of the coarse grass that a horse will reject.

Harrowing the field when the weather is hot and dry is a very useful way of killing parasitic larvae as it exposes them to the sun. Don't do it when it is wet as that simply spreads infective larvae all over the pasture.

Resting a field is another very good method of reducing levels of parasites on pasture, but to be effective it has to be rested for at least six months – a year would be better – which may not be practical in many situations. However, turning out in a field that has been cut for hay can be very effective, especially if the animals are de-wormed twenty-four hours prior to them moving in.

When a new horse moves into communal grazing it should be de-wormed at least twenty-four hours before it is introduced into the field. Use either five consecutive days of Panacur Guard or one dose of Equest, followed the next day with a double dose of tapeworm treatment. In this way you should have ensured as much as possible that a previously incorrectly wormed horse should not contaminate a carefully managed paddock.

To sum up

You will by now have realised there is no such thing as a worm-free horse or pony, and that no single wormer can control all the internal parasites of the animal. By using wormers correctly at the right time and dose, coupled with effective pasture management, you will go a long way to keeping your horse healthy and in peak condition in the most cost-effective way.

One last hint: owners are very bad at estimating the weight of their animals, especially ponies. It is very common to find that while a pony may have been given the correct worming drug it may well have been underdosed. If in doubt use a measuring band, which can be bought for very little at most tack shops. They are not wonderfully accurate but will give you some idea.

CHAPTER FOUR

How Feeding Correctly Can Save You Money

Are you feeding too much?

'You are what you eat' is a well-known adage that is applied to people, but is equally true when talking of horses, or indeed any livestock. There are so many conditions that can be induced by faulty feeding. The most common fault of any equine feeding regime is overfeeding. Time spent thinking about the correct diet for your horse or pony and taking advice from an expert is well worth the effort involved and can save you lots of money – not only in reduced feed bills but in vet fees as well. Your animal is much more likely to stay healthy on a good diet.

Advice on feeding can often be obtained free of charge. Your vet will be able to help, and if necessary refer you to an expert on nutrition. Many feed companies employ nutritionists who, although their advice may well be directed toward their company products, will nonetheless give sound advice in general terms. Do make sure, however, that the 'expert' you consult is properly qualified and not a glorified salesperson.

Let's get down to basics. The horse has evolved over millions of years to be a herd animal that grazes in short bursts and moves on. Even today a horse in a field will spend at least sixty per cent of the time eating. A stabled animal, no matter the diet, only about forty per cent; the rest of the time it's probably getting bored and developing stable vices.

The horse's natural diet is forage, and by that I mean **grass** in the grazing season and hay in

> The most common fault of any equine feeding regime is OVER-FEEDING.

the winter months. These are the best and most natural energy sources. The horse has a highly developed hind gut called the caecum, which has millions of 'good bacteria'. These allow the animal to utilise and ferment large quantities of plant fibre (grass and hay), which is the horse's natural food and forms its basic maintenance diet. Most ponies and many horses, providing that they are not in hard work, will survive and do very well on good quality hay alone as long as they have adequate shelter during inclement weather, and, if not a native pony with a good thick coat, are well rugged up.

If the horse has work to do, as most have, then an adequate diet should be formulated to take the amount

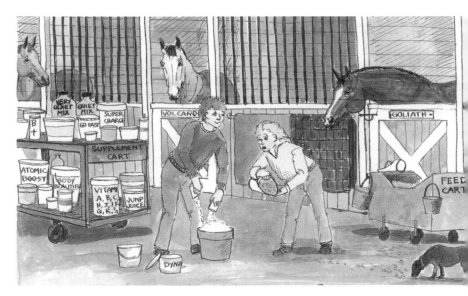

'Where do I put the grain?'

> One of the most distressing sights I see all too often is an overweight animal with laminitis.

of work into account. Most of the time owners will do this on a very *ad hoc* basis, putting in a little of this and more of that, without realising that by so doing they could be mixing two or three perfectly good rations and making one bad feed. It is often so much better to buy feed from one source and to follow the manufacturer's recommendations. Only alter these if the animal is losing or gaining weight or not performing properly, and only then on the advice of your vet.

Laminitis – painfully all too common

One of the most distressing sights I see all too often is an overweight animal with laminitis. It is estimated in Britain alone that **every year there are up to 8,000 new acute cases of laminitis and as many as 12,000 suffering the long-term chronic effects of the disease.** Most of these cases are caused by over-feeding, despite the many warnings that are constantly given by vets and many nutrition experts. It is not only novice horse keepers that fail to heed the warnings. Many 'expert' horse owners who keep their animals for show purposes are prone to over-feed to keep the animals in 'show condition', which in my view just means **fat**.

Laminitis is most common in the spring and is caused by the animal having too much lush, green grass, but it can happen at any time as the result of over-feeding. Left to its own devices the horse or pony – and ponies are far more susceptible to laminitis – will, like any human glutton, live to eat and never know when to stop for its own good. It's the owner's job to try and ensure that the opposite is the case and that it only eats to live and perform.

The lamina is the soft tissue within the foot which connects the pedal bone to the inside of the hoof. It is a highly vascular and sensitive structure and the term 'laminitis' just means inflammation of these tissues. Laminitis occurs when the blood supply to the foot becomes interrupted. Arterial blood is shunted directly into the veins without going through the sensitive lamina, often with disastrous results. Within a very short period of time permanent damage can be done to the foot due to the lack of oxygenated blood. If the disruption to the blood supply is severe and goes on for some time it will affect most of the laminar tissue, and the attachment between the hoof wall and the pedal bone will fail. This will result in either tilting or sinking of the pedal bone. In the very worst cases if the bone keeps descending, it will push through the sole and the animal may have to be put down on welfare grounds. However, even in the worst cases if the correct treatment is given in time – within a few hours of onset of the symptoms – the animal can be saved.

The clinical signs of acute laminitis are all too apparent. It can have a sudden onset and is usually the front feet that are involved. Characteristically the animal rocks back onto its hind legs and tries to put all the weight-bearing onto the heels. There is a strong digital pulse and the feet are usually warm to the touch, although this feature can often misguide a novice owner. The patient will be most reluctant to walk on hard ground but if allowed to stand on a soft surface will be visibly more comfortable. Chronic laminitis is more often seen than the acute form. There is a varying degree of lameness with the pony trying to keep weight on the heels or shifting weight constantly from one foot to the other. It may also look like a 'rocking horse' as it tries to take as much of its weight on the hind legs as possible. There will be rings around the walls of the foot, which are more obvious than the grass rings associated with a change in diet. The soles will be dropped and often convex due to the pedal bone dropping and rotating.

The treatment of laminitis is best left to the vet but if you suspect your horse has the condition, please get professional help as soon as possible. Until the vet arrives, stop feeding grain in any form and do not allow your horse to eat any more grass. The only safe diet to give until the vet advises otherwise, is hay. Do not hose the feet with cold water. It does not help – in fact it has been proved to make the condition worse. Warm water would be more helpful. Don't force the animal to walk unless it is a very short distance to allow it to stand on a soft, thick bed, which will make it more comfortable.

There is a whole armoury of drugs and treatments available to your vet for the treatment of the condition, but many cases will require surgical resection of the hoof wall to relieve pressure and corrective shoeing with heart bar shoes. These are surgical shoes, which should not be fitted until X-rays are taken to determine the exact position of the pedal bone within the foot.

Treatment for laminitis can be very prolonged and painful for both patient and owner. The expense can be considerable and I have known numerous cases costing many hundreds of pounds and the animal left with permanently damaged feet or worst still – dead, as it had to be destroyed to stop further suffering.

> **Treatment for laminitis can be very prolonged and painful for both patient and owner.**

One of the most important attributes of a skilled horse keeper is to be able to retain the animal at a healthy weight. You should be able to feel a horse's or pony's ribs easily without being able to see them. The animal should not have a thick, cresty neck – this is all fat! It is, however, possible to have an otherwise slim animal but with a fat neck and it is possible to get rid of this without emaciating the pony. A mixture of alfalfa and straw, which is commercially available as Dengie HiFi, is very effective as a diet for ponies. A fat Shetland pony would need only about 1.25 lbs of Hi Fi along with about 2 lb of hay twice a day. Fat ponies need to be dieted – not starved.

It can be very difficult to manage some native ponies at grass during the growing season of spring and in the autumn. This is especially true if they are being kept as ornaments and do no work at all. 'Starvation paddocks', where there is very little grass to be obtained, can be part of the answer. They can be partitioned off easily by using an electric fence, but if this is not feasible try fitting a muzzle. These should have a grid at the bottom of the muzzle to enable the animal to drink and nibble whatever grass it can reach. If a muzzle is used, though, do try and make sure that there is nothing in the field on which the animal can become hooked. Old bath taps are especially dangerous.

The golden rule to remember – **unless most horses and all ponies are in hard work, they do not need hard feed at all** and will perform very well on a forage diet.

Problems with youngstock

Over-feeding the growing horse or pony can contribute to problems in the developing bones and joints. Overweight yearlings that do not receive a good balanced diet containing the correct blend of vitamins and minerals, can be very vulnerable to limb deformities, epiphysitis and contracted tendons. Most common among the joint conditions is **osteochondritis dissecans** (OCD), where damage to the lining in a joint can result in small pieces of cartilage becoming separated from the joint surface. The animal becomes chronically lame, and the problem can only be resolved by surgically removing the offending piece of cartilage. Having assisted an orthopaedic veterinary surgeon, I can testify that it is a very skilled and delicate operation using key-hole surgery. Without the operation the animal would remain lame and develop severe arthritis. Many make good recoveries after surgery and have a healthy active lifestyle, but these operations, costing as much as £1,000 depending on the degree of complexity, are still essentially salvage operations. The joint will never be completely healthy and arthritis will inevitably follow at some stage in the animal's life. How much easier and cheaper it is to get the diet right in the first place.

Colic – can you avoid it?

One of the most common causes of colic, which we see every winter, is the constipated horse or pony. The scenario is almost always the same – through boredom or gluttony the horse has been eating its straw bed. The symptoms are not usually violent, although they can become so if left too long untreated. The obvious sign initially, which should ring alarm bells, is a reduction in the normal output of dung which has to be cleared from the stable in the morning. The appetite will diminish to almost nothing and the water container will not have been touched. The patient will be a bit uncomfortable – getting up and lying down – with the bedding churned up for good effect.

A typical case came my way two years ago at Christmas, which is never good timing! A client had left her beloved cob in the care of a good friend. She had left many instructions (and my telephone number) but despite this, on Christmas morning, the inevitable happened. The cob got colic. The cause was easily diagnosed – constipation – and the reason was all too apparent.

His exercise had diminished while the owner was away and, although his feed had been reduced accordingly, he was bored and probably hungry and had eaten his bed. He was very bunged up. Not only was his rectum and colon full of dry, impacted material, but also there seemed to be a fair amount in the caecum as well, which I know can be – from past bitter experience – very difficult to shift.

He was given a large dose of a pain-relieving drug, and by stomach tube liquid paraffin and a salt-water solution. I had to visit him three more times that day and evening – bear in mind it was Christmas Day – as both the 'loco parentis' and I were very concerned about him. It was a round trip of about twenty miles and each time he had to have more injections and fluids until he slowly, oh so slowly, got rid of his burden. Boxing Day finally arrived to find the cob had at long last cleared himself and there was a satisfying pile of dung in one corner and a further mess halfway up the wall!

It was hard to say who had the biggest smile on their face – the horse or horse keeper – and I was quite pleased myself as I was beginning to think only a stick of dynamite would do the job.

The whole unfortunate saga could so easily have been prevented by not bedding on straw in the first place or (if that is not possible) by feeding a bran

> Fed once or twice as a mash, bran can be invaluable in preventing constipation and colic.

mash for a day or two rather than the normal ration. Note that bran should not be fed on a daily basis as part of a ration as it has a mineral imbalance that can be harmful, especially to the growing horse. Fed once or twice as a mash it can be invaluable in preventing constipation and colic.

To make a bran mash put 2–4 lbs of bran in a bucket, depending on the size of the recipient. Pour boiling water – and it must be boiling – onto the bran in sufficient quantity to make a good stiff 'porridge' mixture and stir well. Add 1–2 tablespoons of salt, or Epsom salts if very constipated, cover with a piece of material (we use a piece of clean hessian sacking but that is now a very scarce commodity) and leave to steam for about 15 minutes. It then should be cool enough for the horse to eat. The benefits(!) should be seen next day, and if not, the mash meal can be repeated, providing there are no overt signs of colic and the animal is keen to eat and drink. If not, call the vet!

Another cause of colic induced by feed happens at turn-out in the spring, when many animals are let out onto fresh, green grass. The grass passes through very quickly and the horses start passing green cowpat-like dung. This in itself is usually perfectly normal and to be expected, but some do get colic due to a build-up of excess gas in the system, and they can look like uncomfortable barrage balloons until the symptoms are relieved.

To avoid this happening, limit the time the animal is on the fresh grass to begin with, to allow its digestive system time to get used to the new conditions. It is also a good idea to try and ensure it has had a good feed of hay to fill it up before it goes out, as this not only will make it less hungry but also will tend to reduce the effect of the grass.

All choked up?

One of the many equine conditions which causes owners to panic, is a **choking** horse. To be fair, it can look quite dramatic. Invariably the animal looks utterly miserable. The head and neck are usually extended and stretched straight out. Food and saliva are frequently seen pouring down the nostrils. When the animal coughs, even more material is expelled and the effect can be quite spectacular to an owner who has not seen the condition before.

Choking is caused by an obstruction of the gullet (oesophagus), which is the food passage from the throat to the stomach. Food material is the usual cause of the obstruction and the most common culprit is dried sugar-beet pulp, although other materials such as carrots and apples mixed in feed, if not chewed properly and swallowed too quickly, can cause a problem.

A choke in a horse, although alarming, is not an immediate life-threatening disorder, unlike in cattle and sheep. In ruminants, a choked gullet means that the animal cannot expel gas from the rumen, which is its fourth stomach. This rapidly causes bloat, and pressure from the abdomen due to the accumulated gas results in heart failure; the beast will die in agony within a few short hours if the gas is not released quickly.

Fortunately for the horse, this does not happen as the main organ of digestion (the caecum) is placed further down the gut. Any gas in the system is expelled out of the rear end. The main risk to a horse or pony's health is through dehydration if the blockage is prolonged, as the animal, although prepared to drink, cannot get the fluid into the stomach where it is required. It is possible as well that food material and saliva which is being expelled from the blocked gullet could possibly find its way into the windpipe and cause aspiration pneumonia. This type of pneumonia is very severe, difficult to treat and often fatal. There is also a risk if something hard, like a stick or branch, has been swallowed (it has been known!) that the gullet could be pierced or ruptured, which can have very serious consequences.

Most owners are now well aware of the dangers of feeding dry sugar-beet pulp and the most recent cases I have encountered have involved horses that have broken into food stores and helped themselves.

Fortunately all the horses with blocked gullets that I have seen over the years have got better with treatment, although some take a lot longer than others to resolve. In many cases, however, the choke disappears as quickly as it occurs.

Some ponies or horses, if they bolt their food, can panic if some food material – even a small amount – becomes lodged. The muscles of the gullet go into spasm and the animal becomes distressed. When an owner phones for assistance because of a choke I always tell them to take the animal for a walk. This takes the patient's mind off the food blockage, the muscles in the neck relax and the obstruction often clears before the vet arrives. I never 'break the speed limit' to get to a choke for just that reason.

More serious chokes need more active treatment. Many vets, myself included, will often initially give a patient a sedative as well as a muscle-relaxing drug. This usually allows the muscles in the neck to relax enough for the action of the saliva from the mouth to work through the food material and release the obstruction.

Always use fresh water each time to soak food.

Some cases are more difficult and my last experience was a good one to remember, as it required far more active treatment. She was a Welsh cob who had broken into a food store and eaten dried beet pulp as well as other food material. When I examined her I had a feeling her obstruction was going to be a difficult one to relieve. She was looking very distressed, with some very noxious material pouring out of both nostrils.

I started the standard procedure, which was to sedate her with Domosedan. This makes the patient very sleepy and the head drops down to the knees. I then introduced a stomach tube, which proved the obstruction was somewhere in the chest – about the level of the base of the heart. With a funnel in place, water was poured down the tube while the head was raised, which was hard work for the owner holding the head. With the tube full of water, the head was then lowered quickly to knee level and food material was siphoned off as the water left the tube. It was a laborious procedure and it took many gallons of water and two visits, four hours apart, before the blockage was cleared. Both horse and owner were very pleased. It was one of these cases where I had constantly to reassure the owner that the blockage, given time and patience, would move. I also told him of my worst experience, which was with a Shetland pony. The blockage with that greedy little animal took three days to clear and I was beginning to think the obstruction was set in concrete. The pony survived and has lived another eleven years without further trouble.

To avoid food chokes, and potentially large vet bills, damping feed and soaking sugar-beet pulp is essential. In addition feeding three or even four very small feeds, away from other horses, is better for the animal as it will be less inclined to bolt its feed.

One word of warning on soaking sugar-beet. A client some years ago soaked feed as he was

> **To avoid food chokes, damping feed and soaking sugar-beet pulp is essential.**

directed. Unfortunately he did not change the water each time he soaked the food but used the same water in the same tub for about a week. His horse got severe colic and died because the water had fermented like beer. Always use fresh water each time to soak food.

Water, water ... everywhere

It would be invidious to complete this chapter on feeding without mentioning water. About two thirds of a normal-sized horse, which is 500kg in weight, is water. This means that an average animal of that weight consists of over 300 litres of water.

Water is lost from the body in many ways. It is lost through urine and faecal output, through evaporation when the animal breathes, and through sweating when it is exercised. It has been calculated that **a horse in hard work can lose as much as four gallons of water per hour.** It is known that human athletes experience tiredness when they have lost just two per cent of their body water. It is also known from measurements taken on many occasions that some endurance horses can lose up to ten per cent of their body water on a thirty-five mile ride.

Most horse owners will know how vital it is for the horse always to have access to clean, fresh water. Water of poor quality can cause colic and other digestive disorders and stomach upsets. A horse at any competition or show will compete all the better for being allowed to drink small amounts of water, for example in between rounds if it is a show jumper. Endurance horses should if possible be trained to drink electrolytes at intervals during the competition, or, if they won't take electrolytes – ordinary water. They will perform much better and it could make the difference between winning or losing – or at worst having a very exhausted, sick horse on your hands.

Many horses won't drink away from home because they are reluctant to imbibe 'foreign' water, which tastes and smells very different, possibly due to varying chlorine levels. There is a way round this. At home get them used to drinking water with a slightly peppermint taste by adding a little peppermint essence. This flavouring can then be used when away from home to disguise water from a different supply. If nothing else it will save you the bother of taking bulky, heavy containers of water on trips and outings.

If you are on a long journey, stop and allow the horses to rest and to drink just as often as you yourself need the same. Don't drive for hours with quick changes of driver, without giving your passengers a drink. If you do, you will arrive with an equine athlete that is dehydrated and at a distinct disadvantage before the competition even starts.

In the winter months it is especially important to make sure that water drinkers are not frozen over. An animal that goes without a drink for twenty-four hours, even if it is not working, will be at severe risk of colic. Drinking ice-cold water will not normally cause the animal a problem, providing it is not sweating heavily after exercise when it might be better to allow it to drink tepid water only until it has cooled off a bit.

Stables should if possible be equipped with automatic drinkers. These should be checked at least twice a day to ensure they are working correctly and have not been contaminated with faeces or anything else which may deter the animal from drinking. Fresh water should be available at all times in the stable or paddock. It is vital to the horse's health and well-being.

Money and time ensuring a good constant supply of fresh clean water will pay dividends in reduced vet bills.

CHAPTER FIVE

The Environment – Get it Right and Keep Your Cash

Stabling – won't any old shed do?

It's only a personal opinion, but it is my belief that horses are not nearly so well housed as they used to be in Victorian and Edwardian times. Look around any stately home – and many others that were not so stately, like the local doctor's or vicarage – and have a look at what used to be the stables. Notice the height of the roof. Look at how well constructed the drains were, with seemingly no expense spared. Look at the space that was designated to each animal. In many establishments the horses were of course in stalls, but the general level of care and horse management was in very many instances streets ahead of that seen in modern yards.

Take a long, hard look at your horse accommodation or, even better, get a knowledgeable person to cast a critical eye over it. Points that should be considered are many but these in particular spring to mind.

Is the floor in good condition or is the surface in poor repair even although it is conveniently hidden from view under the straw? It does seem rather obvious that the surface on which the animal stands should be as clean, dry and as slip-free as possible.

In the very worst stabling incident with which I was involved, some idiot had actually built a stable over a cesspit, with the man-hole cover in the middle of the stable floor. Whoever it was that perpetrated this folly then sold the property to someone else who gave the matter no thought whatsoever until one fateful day when a 16.2hh thoroughbred put one hind foot and then the other through the rusting iron cover. When the fire brigade and I arrived the horse was stuck up to its hips in the hole and could not move. The smell from the pit below was horrendous, and the prospect of getting the animal out injury-free did not look very encouraging. We tried all sorts of ways to release the horse to no avail, until I realised that the only way was to remove the roof, put a harness on the beast and hoist it out with the help of a JCB. It took about two hours altogether to effect the rescue. In the end all was well and the horse came away with only superficial injuries. It was very lucky indeed. As for the stable, it was halfway demolished getting to the beast and then completely knocked down on my instructions before I left.

Many modern custom-built stable blocks look very smart but have very poor ventilation. There is a commonly held belief that if a stable has a half door this will give the animal enough fresh air. It does not. The air at the back of the box may not be circulating and be very unhealthy, especially if the roof is too low (and often it is). (There's more about ventilation later in this chapter.)

There should be enough space in the stable to allow the horse to move around with as low a risk as possible of the horse becoming cast.

Drainage too can be a problem. If the drainage is bad, no matter how absorbent the bedding, it may become saturated and result in all sorts of foot infections. Wet bedding will also raise the humid-

> There is a commonly held belief that if a stable has a half door this will give the animal enough fresh air. It does not.

ity in the atmosphere, which, if the ventilation is poor, will increase the levels of bacteria and fungal spores in the air (this is discussed in more detail later in this chapter). This can be exacerbated if the mucking-out is less than diligent.

Carefully **inspect all the surfaces of the box for any sharp projections** such as nails or bolts. I have lost count of the number of times I have been called to stitch lacerated lips and torn noses caused by just such protrusions. Less obvious as a hazard is the glass in the window or a ceramic sink used as a feeding basin. A horse I used to know died as the result of kicking at a white butler-style sink whose sides had not been adequately protected. The sink was shattered and a long, very thin shard of the material completely cut through the tendons of the right hind leg. The animal was not insured and was put down as the injury had effectively put an end to its working life. Simple measures to remove potential hazards can save you heartache and money.

The vice squad

Remember that horses are naturally herd animals. They are not solitary creatures and like to be part of a group. Domestication can mean for many that they are kept for long, lonely hours in a stable or even isolated in a remote paddock without sight or sound of a fellow creature. Boredom, in addition to separation anxiety, is all too common, especially after the animal has eaten its ration of feed. It is hardly surprising, given these facts, that many horses and ponies become very stressed and develop stable vices.

Common vices include aimless **box walking** or **weaving**, crib-

> Boredom, in addition to separation anxiety, is all too common.

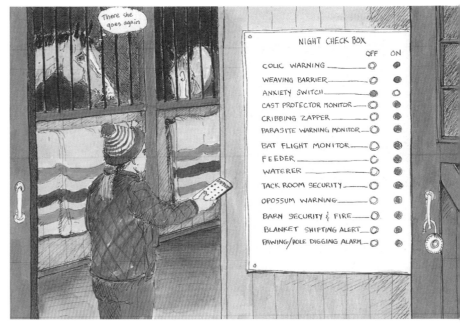

'Good night, boys. I'll be back to check on you soon.'

biting (wood chewing), which usually leads to **wind-sucking**, **head-nodding** and, in very extreme situations, **self-mutilation**.

It is vital to check neurotic behaviour before it gets well established as it can be very difficult, or even impossible, to eradicate, even when the cause of the behaviour is remedied.

Crib-biting and wind-sucking (where in most cases the animal fixes its teeth on any horizontal surface, bites and then flexes its neck and takes in air with a grunt) almost always starts in the stable. This pattern of behaviour can be learned from other horses and will only be seen in the field if it has been learned in the stable.

Controlling the vice is not easy as some horses can wind-suck without the need to crib-bite, but is usually aimed at reducing the surfaces on which the animal can chew. The manger should be removed and a metal strip placed along the open stable door. Cover all the other surfaces with a non-toxic noxious material. Commercial products are readily available for this if old-fashioned creosote doesn't work. Wind-sucking, which is often thought to be very harmful to the horse because it can cause it to lose condition, can be controlled by a leather strap around the top of the neck. This seems to work by stopping the animal from arching its neck.

Weaving from side to side and box walking are both symptoms of anxiety and chronic boredom. If prolonged, both types of behaviour will result in damage to feet, tendons and ligaments. Weaving over an open door can be stopped by means of a V-shaped grille placed over the door. All sorts of means can be used to alleviate boredom. Commercial toys are available, and the most successful I have seen is a rubber ball suspended from the roof, and a large swede or turnip similarly attached for the horse to chew on.

What nervous and stressed animals most require is **company**, such as a goat or small pony. One of the best show jumpers I have ever known used to travel the show-jumping circuit with a goat for company. One day the goat did not come with him – I don't know why – and the animal almost demolished the breeze-block wall in the competition stables. When the goat was with him he was subdued, quiet and settled in the box.

Box walking, or pacing as it can also be known, can be very harmful to the horse especially if it is shut in for medical reasons. This is often the case for a horse with damaged tendons. One of my clients with just this problem found a very effective way to stop the boredom. She bought a large, empty, plastic beer barrel, the type that is often used for making home-brewed beer. It was a fairly robust structure – purchased from Boots, the chemists – and she cut several holes in its sides. It was then part-filled with pony nuts, and the horse quickly realised that by rolling the vessel around it could, with some difficulty, extract the feed over a few hours. The animal had to box rest for a number of weeks and this simple device worked well for him.

Considering how most horses and ponies are kept, it is surprising that stable vices are not more common than they are. These stresses can be avoided with care, thought and often little expense, but there is no doubt that the best remedy in the long run is to allow them as far as possible to be as nature intended – running free in a social group.

Fresh air – it's essential and it's free!

Poor ventilation is the single most common fault to be found in any form of stabling. Ideally air should be encouraged to enter the building at about head height and to leave through the roof. However, there are variations on this ideal, such as louvred windows (without glass) at or above head level which can be adjusted to cope with prevailing weather conditions. But before you start cutting holes in your stable it may be wise to get some expert advice on the matter from your vet. Most experienced vets will be able to spot the good and bad points very quickly, and simple remedial measures may be very effective in countering respiratory disease. Remember, though: there is a fine dividing line between creating a good, fresh environment and a draught.

One of the most significant respiratory conditions which

> **Poor ventilation is the single most common fault to be found in any form of stabling.**

affects horses and ponies, and which is especially common during the later winter months of February and March, is **chronic obstructive pulmonary disease (COPD)**. This is an asthma-like condition caused by an allergic reaction within the respiratory passages to fungal spores and dust from hay and straw.

In the mild form of the disease, the patient may have only an occasional dry, hacking cough. This is often heard when the animal is feeding or after some light exercise. There may also be a persistent, thin, grey nasal discharge. If your horse or pony has these symptoms then beware. It is a warning signal. The animal could at any time develop severe respiratory distress, which used to be known as 'broken wind' or 'heaves'.

On at least two occasions in the last three years I have been called to horses with what their owners described as colic symptoms. The patients were all breathing heavily and in great distress, as if in pain. However, as I listened to the lungs it was apparent from the harsh sounds coming through the stethoscope that they were suffering very badly from COPD.

Diagnosis of the condition is usually straightforward but is made more difficult by the possible presence of respiratory infection. Many veterinary practices now use flexible endoscopes to look down the windpipe of problem cases, where it is possible to see 'pools of pus' in the lung passages, when infection is a complicating feature of the disease.

> **Prevention of COPD is so much cheaper than treatment, and it's something you can do yourself for your horse.**

Treatment of the disease has to be left to the vet but can be expensive depending on the severity of the disease. The most common drug used for treatment is Ventipulmin, a tub of which can cost as much as filling a car full of petrol. Severe breathing difficulties have to be treated with intravenous drugs which, if they have to be repeated for a few days, will quickly push the costs into hundreds of pounds.

Prevention of COPD is all-important and so much cheaper than treatment, and it's something you can do yourself for your horse.

Fresh air is the vital requirement. For many horses and ponies with the chronic form of the condition the only remedy that works in the winter months is to turn them out in a New Zealand rug. They should have access to a field shelter, which will protect them from the worst of the wind and rain, but will allow free passage of air. If this is not possible and the animal has to be stabled, then it should be kept on shavings, peat or a paper bed, with good under-drainage to ensure a dust-free environment. If hay is to be fed it must be soaked first and then allowed to drain. Soaking with a bucket of water or turning a hose onto a net of hay does not work. It must be totally immersed in water for between 30 and 60 minutes to allow the water to cause the fungal spores to swell and de-nature. If hay is soaked longer, and some owners do this overnight, it will lose much of its feed value and become unpalatable.

Another, often better, alternative to hay is high-fibre feed such as haylage or Dengie Hi Fi. But remember – please – **it is pointless to feed your horse correctly if the one next door in the same air space is eating unsoaked hay and is bedded on straw.**

Another common fault is storing hay next door to a stable block into which fungal spores can blow directly when the wind is in the right direction.

A stable must be looked at critically and if it is covered in cobwebs, as so many are, these must be removed and all dust particles with them. This can be done with an industrial vacuum cleaner or with a power hose. **Never ignore a dry cough**. It could mean that your horse or pony may become acutely ill at any time, but if you apply simple measures to the environment you could save your pocket and your horse much distress.

The outdoor life – the healthy option?

Living out of doors is naturally more healthy for horses and ponies, and all equines, if they could talk, would I am sure tell you they would much prefer to be out in a paddock than inside a stable.

This does not mean you can sit back and relax knowing your animal is in the fresh air and can come to no harm. Having just talked about **winter COPD** and extolling the virtues of fresh air, it now seems a little perverse to talk about **summer COPD**, which is the result of breathing fresh air but contaminated with pollen.

It is quite common for horses which have tendencies towards winter COPD and need to live outside in those months, to have very similar symptoms in the summer when the pollen counts are high. The pollen mostly comes from grass and trees but some horses are very sensitive to rape-seed pollen. Like people, horses often show hypersensitivity to more than one agent.

The symptoms of summer COPD are very similar to those of the disease in winter. In the early stages the patient will have an intermittent cough, which is harsh, dry and unproductive. There is an increase in the respiratory rate, which initially is slight. The normal rate for the horse at rest is 8-10 breaths per minute. This can be easily checked by simple observation as you hang over the stable door or field gate. If you find the animal is consistently breathing faster than normal and it has a dry cough, then this could well mean that it is beginning to suffer from COPD. However, do remember that if the weather is hot, and especially if it is humid as well, the respiratory rate may be enhanced, and that this is as normal as breathing faster during and after exercise.

Prevention of summer COPD is not easy. Pollen is everywhere, and although a pollen count will be reduced in a bare, windswept paddock with no natural trees or hedges for cover, it is no guarantee that a pollen-affected horse will not be at risk.

One client with a pollen-affected animal stabled the horse during the day and allowed it out to graze at night. This strategy seemed to work initially and then its breathing became very distressed again. I was called out and found the horse being kept in a barn with good ventilation but in the next-door box was a load of hay bales that had only recently been brought in from the hay field. This animal had no previous history of winter COPD, but I was sure that the new hay was the reason why stabling the animal had suddenly made the condition worse. The only immediate solution was to turn the patient out again through the day until the barn was cleared and cleaned. This, coupled with a change of treatment, improved the breathing within a few hours.

Another condition of the outdoor summer months, which is very difficult to treat and fathom, is **head shaking**. It is a very poorly understood syndrome, which seems to affect horses far more commonly than ponies. It can make a riding horse extremely intractable and difficult – if not impossible and dangerous – to ride.

A case I dealt with just this year started in March/April time. The affected animal is a ten-year-old mare, which during the previous year had started twitching her head from side to side when being ridden. This year the condition got worse as the season went on, producing vigorous up and down movements of the head. Finally the mare resorted to holding her head very close to the ground, but as soon the she stopped moving she resumed a perfectly normal demeanour and behaved herself (apart from a tendency to rub her nose against either of her front legs). The problem would be severe on some days but, seemingly without rhyme or reason, almost non-existent on others.

Over the years many horses have undergone thorough investigations in an effort to try and identify the cause of head shaking. The eyes are examined for abnormalities, and an endoscope (a fibre optic instrument) is employed to look up the nostrils and at the back of the throat – this is to check for signs of infection, tumours or for allergic reactions. Radiographs may also be taken, but in most animals these have produced little by way of a positive result. Some believe it worthwhile to check inside the ears, as ear infections, especially if there are mites in the ear canal, can cause intense irritation. Another possible source is an abscess at the base of a tooth – and everyone knows just how painful toothache can be. It is also possible that a horse is just irritated beyond measure by poorly fitting tack.

I tried all these avenues with this ten-year-old mare but, as on so many occasions in the past, with negative results.

I used to think that most idiopathic (unknown origin) head shakers were reacting to insects or flies in their environment, but in recent times I have revised this theory and this particular patient influenced me in this opinion.

Working on the basis that the nasal passages were being irritated by pollen – in a way similar to hay fever in people – I recommended that the owner tried a muzzle net. This is a product that has been researched and used in the USA. Clinical trials have shown that eighty per cent of horses with these symptoms evince measurable improvements with a muzzle net, which works by excluding (at best) or reducing the levels of pollen entering the nostrils. The mask certainly helped with this case although it was not one hundred per cent effective.

Other cases of head shaking may be caused by sensitivity to light, which is again not incompatible with the pollen theory as human sufferers of hay fever will testify. For those cases a form of horse sunglasses can now be used. Again these were first marketed in America but are now available in Britain, and I am told they are very effective and relatively inexpensive to buy. Another client tried both the masks and shades and was very pleased with the results.

If you have a problem 'head shaker' and have eliminated the very obvious causes such as tack or teeth, it may be cost-effective to try the mask or shades, before embarking on very expensive diagnostic tests, which all too often prove very little.

The perfect paddock
Ideally in the summer a stocking rate of one horse per three acres is ideal and should not be less than **one acre per animal**. A small paddock if grazed continually very soon becomes 'horse sick'. This means the grass will look very unappetising and coarse, especially where the droppings have not been picked up, and the ground may look very bare and poached.

All paddocks should have a source of fresh water preferably supplied automatically in a trough and not a stagnant pond or smelly ditch which could be contaminated with all sorts of potential pathogens. If the water source is a river, it should not have steep banks, which might be hazardous to the animal going down or coming back from having a drink. The fire brigade and I have spent too much time extracting horses from drains and rivers for me to be comfortable with horses drinking from rivers.

Gates and fences should be checked to be sure they are in good repair. Barbed wire should never be allowed in a paddock or field that grazes horses. Electric fences can be useful and non-hazardous for temporary fencing and when used to stop horses from leaning through or over wooden rails to get to 'the greener grass on the other side'. Debris such as broken jumping poles or even farm machinery must be cleared away as these can be very dangerous to an animal having a mad moment, as most do from time to time.

For a horse an ideal field should have ample grazing, at least one companion and some form of natural shelter (even in the summer) such as a hedge or leafy tree to provide some protection against the elements of rain, wind or heat.

Unfortunately, all too often this is not the case. Many fields which are otherwise suitable are contaminated by poisonous plants, which are a significant serious threat to the horse population.

The yellow peril

Yellow is a bright, happy colour. In the spring it means daffodils and forsythia. In the summer we see buttercups in the pasture, and fields with oilseed rape splash yellow all over the landscape. Unfortunately, there is another all too common summer plant which has a yellow flower that is the cause of much distress to many horses and owners – **ragwort**, or, to give it its proper botanical name, *Senecio jacobaea*.

Ragwort is a weed and it grows everywhere, despite (in Britain) a law (which is never enforced) which makes it an offence to allow ragwort to grow unhindered on your land. At one time landlords were fined for not keeping ragwort under control.

> **Acute ragwort poisoning is not too common, but chronic ragwort poisoning IS.**

The plant contains an alkaloid, pyrrolizidine, which causes severe damage to liver cells and results in liver failure. This failure can be acute, with a very sudden onset, or chronic, where the animal gradually loses weight and condition.

I have seen many cases of acute ragwort poisoning over the years and almost all have occurred in the spring when the horses have been on virtually bare earth paddocks. Then the only bit of greenery that is coming through the soil is the ragwort plant and many horses and ponies will, when it is emerging like this and there is nothing else to nibble, eat it with disastrous consequences.

I had one case a few years ago that I was called to at about ten o'clock at night. The animal – it was only about three years old – had crashed over a railway line and barged through a barbed-wire fence. It was oblivious to everything due to acute hepatic encephalopathy. It was aimlessly wandering, blind, and inclined to be aggressive as well. I did not need a blood sample to confirm the diagnosis. One look at the paddock on which it had been grazing, coupled with the clinical symptoms it was showing, was enough to decide that it had to be put out of its misery as quickly as possible.

Thankfully, acute poisoning is not too common. However, chronic ragwort poisoning is. Up to ten cases a year will be seen by myself or one of my colleagues and many others must go undiagnosed. The chronic disease is almost certainly the result of eating the plant dry in hay over a period of time, when it is relatively palatable. I have never seen horses or ponies eating the adult mature plant while it is growing. It is very bitter, but when it is dried and in hay and often difficult to distinguish from a dried thistle, it will be eaten without too much difficulty.

The symptoms of chronic poisoning are non-specific and can be attributed to other diseases. Commonly the animal will lose weight and have a poor appetite. There may be some diarrhoea and photosensitisation (sunburn) and later, signs of jaundice and fluid retention along the belly. A blood sample will confirm the diagnosis, and if the animal is not too severely ill, treatment may be attempted.

This initially must be left to the vet as there is no specific treatment for liver failure, but high doses of multivitamins and a high carbohydrate diet may prove helpful. The liver is one of the few organs in the body, which can regenerate itself to some extent, and, providing the damage is not too severe, I have known some animals to recover from chronic poisoning.

About a month ago I had to put an old pony to sleep because of chronic hepatopathy, the result – almost certainly – of eating ragwort over a period of time, perhaps even years. It was getting thinner by the day and losing interest in eating. It had been on extra feed and vitamins, the teeth had been rasped flat and a fortune paid for worming doses. However, the blood sample revealed the true cause of the malaise. I had to advise that in this case, unfortunately, the damage was too severe and the prospect of recovery almost nil. It was put down. As I did the job I glanced at the younger stable mate who looked very well and hoped that the hard lesson had been learned and that it would be safe from the effects of the weed.

Ragwort is very difficult to eradicate. Chemicals will do the job and can be expensive, but what price do you put on the safety of your horse?

The other, cheaper method is hard work. Ragwort is difficult to dig up or pull out of the ground.

> **Check your field thoroughly for poisonous plants, remembering just how far horses and ponies can reach over a fence.**

Weeding by hand must be done (use gloves!) before the plant begins to seed or it is a waste of time. Burn it after weeding to destroy it completely.

If you are buying hay, try to check it for suspicious-looking plants and if in any doubt remove them from the hay. Even better, if you know which field is to be cut for hay, check it for the noxious weed before the grass is cut. Yes, I know this involves time and hard work, but it could cut down on vets' bills and save your animal's life.

Whilst ragwort is the most common source of poison to the horse, many others exist. **Yew** is deadly. One mouthful will kill, so you must ensure that your animal cannot stretch across a fence to reach the tree, and that no one throws tree or hedge clippings into the horse's field.

Common plants such as **privet** or even **buttercups**, which can look so nice in a pasture, can be poisonous if eaten in sufficient quantity. Many others including **rhododendron**, **oleander**, **foxglove** and **deadly nightshade** are rarely eaten but can be poisonous. This is by no means meant to be a definitive list of poisonous plants.

Check your field thoroughly for plants, remembering just how far horses and ponies can reach over a fence. If you are in doubt about any plant or weed consult a textbook or take a sample to your vet. **But if in doubt – pull it out!**

CHAPTER SIX

For Want of a Nail ...

The importance of good shoeing

Most lameness problems originate in the foot, and you may be surprised to read that often they can be the result of poor shoeing. Do you know if your farrier is doing a good job, or do you just leave it up to him?

In recent studies it has been proved that **up to ninety-five per cent of all horses have some form of foot imbalance** (*No Foot, No Horse,* Williams and Deacon, Kenilworth Press), which can dispose them to all manner of injury. In truth, if the foot is not prepared correctly (i.e. well balanced), the horse can suffer repercussions in the joints of his feet and legs, and possibly right up to his shoulders, neck and back.

If you thought the above statistic was alarming, try these two: **up to seventy per cent of horses that are in work in one year have a muscle or tendon injury, and in over seventy-five per cent of these horses the lameness was the result of or was contributed to by bad shoeing or feet trimming.**

A badly prepared foot will mean that the animal's limb structure is off balance. When exercising, this may cause it to over-compensate and pull or tear a ligament or tendon. A badly balanced foot can also cause a horse to develop a poor stride pattern or gait, which may lead to the animal injuring itself while in motion. A simple injury such as over-reaching, where the toe of the hind foot hits the heels of the front foot, or forging, where it hits the front sole can be caused by tiredness, but it can also be caused by the toes being too long.

> **Up to ninety-five per cent of all horses have some form of foot imbalance.**

Take the trouble to learn about this important aspect of horse care – it really could save you a small fortune.

Here are a number of simple criteria you can apply which will give you some idea whether you have cause for concern or not.

Firstly, the front feet should be identical to each other in shape and size. The same applies to the back feet. Back feet, as a general rule, are longer and narrower than the front feet.

With the horse standing squarely on all four feet on a level surface carefully look at the front feet from the side. (Here comes the technical bit.) Draw an imaginary line through the pastern and continue that through the hoof. That line should be continuous and straight, and if there is any deviation in the line it means that the animal has defective hoof/pastern axis and that the foot is unbal-

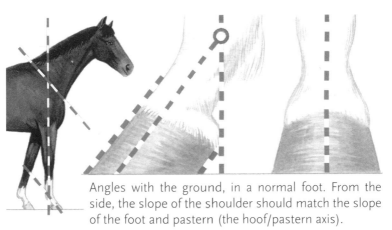

Angles with the ground, in a normal foot. From the side, the slope of the shoulder should match the slope of the foot and pastern (the hoof/pastern axis).

limbs are upright and in alignment

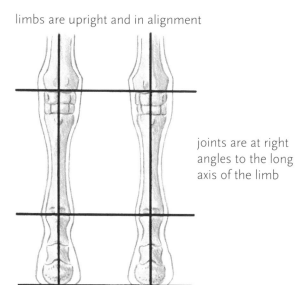

joints are at right angles to the long axis of the limb

A line through the leg should bisect all the joints and the foot.

anced, which puts an incredible strain on the horse when it is moving.

The hoof wall and the heel wall should also be in parallel, and the usual reason for the defective hoof/pastern axis is that the toe has been allowed to grow too long and the heels have collapsed or often – mistakenly – been rasped flat.

Stand in front of the horse and again draw a line down the centre of the cannon bone and continue this line down through the hoof. This line should divide the hoof into two equal parts. If it does not it means the balance between the inside and outside of the foot is wrong. Double-check this by looking at the foot when it is unshod. The heels should be the same height. It is a common fault in many horses that the outside heel is higher than the inside, which throws the foot – and whole horse – out of balance. A farriers' T-square can also be used – see diagram – which will very easily give a good assessment of what is called the foot medio-lateral balance.

If you have done these checks for yourself and feel that you have cause for concern it may be better first to discuss your worries with your vet. The farrier is a professional and may not take kindly to a lay opinion – even if it is correct – as to the quality of his or her work. He will probably be much less resistant to veterinary opinion and many problems can often be rectified at this level. Your vet may be able to do this as one of those 'while you are here' jobs, but give the practice some advance warning so that they send an experienced equine vet, as it may not be fair to subject a new graduate to that type of pressure. If the feet are badly or incorrectly

bearing surface of foot should be parallel to right-angled bar of T-square

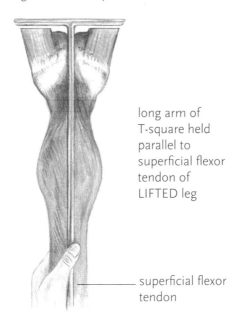

long arm of T-square held parallel to superficial flexor tendon of LIFTED leg

superficial flexor tendon

Checking foot balance with the aid of a farriers' T-square – your farrier can show you how to do this.

shod then the choice is yours to seek a new farrier, but it may pay you to stay with the one you have if he or she is open to taking advice from the vet and is capable and willing to act on it. To do nothing is not an option; your horse will inevitably suffer in the long run.

Shoeing is expensive – why so often?

Horse and pony hooves are like the nails on our hands and feet. Both are made of horny material secreted by the coronary band (in the horse), or by the nail beds (in people). Both are hard but of an elastic material designed to protect sensitive underlying tissue. Everyone knows from personal experience that nails have to be kept regularly trimmed if they are to stay healthy and in good shape. Because equines have to walk and run on their 'nails', it is even more important that regular trimming and shoeing is done every **four to six weeks**. Never be tempted to make the shoeing intervals longer than this. Just because the shoes are still on the feet after six weeks, it does not mean that the feet don't need attention. Far from it. Leaving the shoes on for longer will almost certainly invite problems in the future – problems that could be expensive and put your horse out of work. Even a week can make the difference between the horse going lame, with all the costs that could be involved, or remaining sound.

> It is a common mistake to believe that the unshod horse or pony can be left without farriery care for longer periods than those animals with shoes.

Horses have to be shod to prevent undue wear of the hoof, which would otherwise damage the foot, and also to spread the weight-bearing load around the hoof wall. Unshod horses and ponies can do light work but only

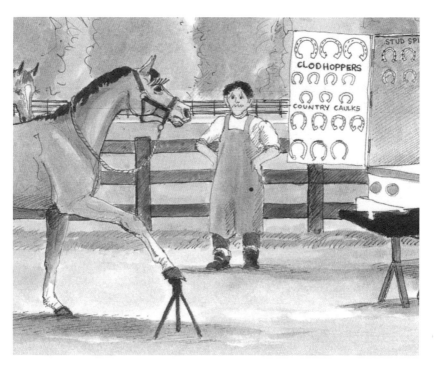

Do you have anything in a wide-webbed pump?

away from hard surfaces, such as roads. It is a common mistake to believe that the unshod horse or pony can be left without farriery care for longer periods than those animals with shoes. This is not the case – **unshod horses must have their feet trimmed at regular intervals** to keep them in good condition.

It is never too early to start a good foot-care regime. Even before it is time for them to be shod youngsters benefit from having their feet checked and trimmed by the farrier once a month. This is just good practical sense as it should ensure the growth of well-shaped feet and the animals will be completely happy with the farrier before they need to have shoes.

The horn in the hoof grows about one centimetre per month (nearly half an inch), although this may vary a little depending on the health and nutritional state of the animal. Again, thinking in human terms, most people will be aware that their own nails reflect their health status. If a person has had a period of illness, their nails will often look very dry and be brittle. Horses' feet are the similar in this respect, but poor quality horn may not be apparent until a few weeks or even months after the animal has been ill or on poor nutrition. It takes between nine to twelve months for new horn to grow down from the coronary band to the weight-bearing surface.

Look after your farrier

Given the statistics that so many horses are lame due to poor foot balance then it stands to reason that there must be many bad farriers at work today. It's a frightening thought! But there are many good, well-qualified farriers in every part of the country. It may make sense to pay that bit extra for a farrier with a justifiably good reputation if it means that your animal's feet are well maintained and shod.

Trimming and balancing the foot is the most important skill a good farrier has to learn and it can take time to do well. Try not to hurry a farrier. Maximise the time that he or she has to spend on the yard by always having the horse ready to be shod and well presented, with the feet picked out and clean. It's wasting your time and money if the farrier has to bang away on an empty anvil while the horse is caught and brought in from the field, and then he has to clean the foot before he can start.

> Do you know if your farrier is doing a good job, or do you just leave it up to him?

A good farrier will want to take time over his work and will be patient with a restless horse. It always pays to look after him if he is doing a good job. The odd cup of coffee (and slice of cake!) after the job is done and the money paid on time will be much appreciated, and it will make it all the more likely that the next visit will be at the time agreed. Make the next appointment for four to six weeks' time before he leaves the yard. That way neither you nor the farrier is likely to forget.

Daily care

The owner has a vital role to play in his or her horse's foot care. Daily care of the feet is simple but very important and could save you huge vet bills.

Feet should be picked out at least twice a day, and the animal should not be allowed to stand around for any length of time in wet, muddy conditions. Stable floors must be well drained and dry underfoot. Caked-on mud should be washed off as this can dry out the hooves and make them brittle. It is still a matter for discussion whether an animal benefits from having the hoof wall oiled, but the current opinion is that while this may make the foot look well cared for and smart, it may also be harmful. The hoof wall is covered by a thin membrane, which controls the movement of moisture into and out of the wall, and if hoof oil is applied regularly it can stop this flow of moisture and may damage the hoof wall.

Abscesses

It is very common to be called to a lame horse and for the owner to proclaim that in their opinion the lameness is in the shoulder. While I never dispute this assertion (well, not to start with anyway!) I always begin an examination at the animal's hoof, as I know very well that a very high percentage of horses are lame due to pain in the foot or the surrounding structures. Abscesses are a case in point.

'Simple things satisfy simple minds' is an old adage I slip into with the greatest ease. I still find it very satisfying to diagnose and treat a foot abscess in the horse or pony, even though it is a very common condition. Foot abscesses seem to be more common in the winter months. This is due to the prevailing weather causing the ground to be wet and muddy, which makes the sole of the animal's foot softer than it would otherwise be and therefore much more liable to penetration and infection. Also, a foot that is sinking deep into mud all day will be by definition very dirty, which gives another good reason why foot abscesses are seen much more commonly in January or February.

Bacteria present in the mud or soil and on the foot can penetrate a puncture wound caused by a nail prick or a sharp stone. Cracks in the foot as the result of neglect by infrequent shoeing or trimming or the hoof wall being brittle will also allow infection to creep up into and under the sole and the result is an abscess.

Clinically, when an infection is starting, the horse may only be slightly lame. At this point, although an abscess may be suspected because the offending foot is warmer than its opposite number, it may still be very difficult to find. As the pus builds up in the hoof, the foot will become very sore and the pain severe enough to stop the animal from eating; it may even refuse to put the foot to the ground. It is often quite common at this stage to find the leg, up to and above the fetlock, swollen with fluid. This is a form of lymphangitis and it is not uncommon for owners to be in fear that their animal has tendon damage, or in local parlance 'done a tendon'.

I still get quite a boost when I remove a shoe, dig into a sole and am rewarded by a thin trickle of grey-black purulent material. It is all the more pleasing if the patient has had a swollen leg and been in great pain and by next morning the swelling has gone down, the pain has almost gone and the animal and owner are smiling again.

If an abscess is not discovered quickly enough and drained down through the foot, pus may track up the foot and emerge at the coronary band. When this happens it is known as a quittor, and this type of infection is much more difficult to clear up.

Once an abscess is discovered, treatment is straight-forward. Good drainage is essential. A hole, just large enough to allow pus to escape easily, is 'dished out', taking care not to damage other adjoining sensitive tissues. The vet or a good farrier ought to do this. Do not attempt it yourself. At this stage the owner can save further visits from the vet by taking over – with the vet's approval – the ongoing treatment.

The foot will have to be poulticed daily for at least two to three days to ensure successful drainage of all the infection from the hoof. Animalintex is commonly used for this purpose, but in the past I have used simple (and cheaper) bran poultices to good effect. I have also heard of bread being used for the same job and that it worked well. Basically any similar material will do providing it will retain warmth and 'draw' the infection.

The poultice should be changed at least once in twenty-four hours, and if for any reason it is not possible to poultice the foot (the patient may not tolerate the foot bandage or bag) then it is possible to stand the limb three to four times a day in a bucket of warm water to which is added a handful of salt or Epsom salts. This is known as 'tubbing' and it helps to draw out purulent material.

> **Delaying the farrier by even a week or two may result in an abscess.**

The vet should ascertain that the horse has been properly protected against tetanus, and, if not, will give immediate temporary cover with tetanus antitoxin. This is vital to protect against tetanus. Antibiotics are almost always given at the same time to help mop up any residual infection.

Prevention of an abscess is always easier and cheaper than a cure as it may take quite a few weeks for the horse to become sound again especially if the infection is very deep seated.

Some horses may develop cracks or splits along the bottom of the hoof during the summer months, which can allow infection into the foot. This is more common in unshod animals, and regular trimming will help to prevent cracking and brittle feet. A delay of even a week or two by the farrier may result in an abscess.

Biotin and methionine supplements – biotin in particular – can be helpful in all-round foot care and maintainence of a healthy foot. Years ago I had a horse that seemed to get an abscess just about every other month – in different feet. After using a biotin supplement (Farrier's Formula) the problem disappeared.

Thrush

Thrush is another type of foot infection which can wholly be prevented by good foot care. It is the result of a bacterial infection in the clefts of the frog, which causes damage to the frog, a very foul smell and lameness. It is easily prevented by good hygiene. This means picking out the feet twice daily, cleaning the clefts of the frog if necessary with a dilute iodine solution, and making sure that the horse has a clean, dry bed to stand on.

Some other common foot problems

Other foot conditions such as **bruised soles** and **corns** can be avoided with care. These conditions are the result of standing on a solid object such as a stone, or by repeated trauma to the sole caused by a poorly fitting shoe (either left on too long or poor farriery), or by too much work on hard ground. Making sure this does not happen can be fairly easy in most horses but more difficult if the animal is flat-footed and thin-soled.

Laminitis is very common, especially in ponies, and owners can do much to stop it happening. The most common cause of the disease is over-eating, and the consequences for the animal can be disastrous. A detailed account of the illness is available in Chapter 4.

Navicular disease

There are some conditions of the foot, which have an unknown aetiology (causation). No one has been able to fully explain why some horses get navicular disease, but I do believe that many cases can or should be preventable with good shoeing. I also believe that poor shoeing over a period of time could be responsible.

Many horses with the disease, or syndrome as it is now fashionable to call it, have poor foot conformation. They commonly have long toes and low, collapsed heels – which can sometimes be the product of defective foot trimming and shoeing – although the condition is also seen in horses with upright, narrow feet (often called 'boxy feet').

As a general practitioner, I find it a lameness that most clients

> I do believe that many cases of navicular disease can or should be preventable with good shoeing.

dread and yet – perversely – they are all too ready to pre-diagnose it for themselves. The problem with the syndrome is that it has many different clinical signs, because there can be multiple causes of pain in the navicular bone giving a range of different presenting features. Unfortunately, the very least that is required to diagnose navicular syndrome is an X-ray machine. Fortunately, however, good, corrective shoeing – to reduce as much as possible the consequences of bad foot balance – can help a great deal to treat the onset of symptoms, and there are drugs that can help too. So it's not all bad news.

The navicular bone lies at the back of the last joint in the foot known as the coffin joint. It is supported by suspensory ligaments, and the deep flexor tendon passes over the back surface of the bone. There have been many theories over the years as to the cause of the 'disease', including a form of arthritis, but impaired blood circulation to the bone and back of the foot now seems to be the most likely culprit.

Navicular syndrome is far more common in horses than in ponies; indeed some textbooks will say it does not occur in ponies. It is also said to affect the front feet only, which does seem to be the case. Initially the stride length tends to be shortened and the animal will have a history of stumbling. Lameness may be accentuated by flexing the fetlock and the lower joints within the foot. Pressure from hoof testers will rarely show pain. Lungeing on a hard, level surface can be very useful as a diagnostic technique. Left foreleg lameness will show on the left rein and right foreleg lameness on the right rein. All these signs are easy to understand and are textbook stuff, but my last case, encountered only the other week, was very different.

The client had, and still has, I'm glad to say, a very

good-looking show pony. The feet were well shod, although the heels were lower than I like to see. The eight-year-old mare had a history of a near foreleg lameness, which could be quite acute and painful. There was nothing obvious on clinical examination, and the owner always declined a lameness work-up with nerve blocks and X-rays as she knew from past experience that after a few days' rest, along with phenylbutazone (which is a commonly used anti-inflammatory and pain-relieving drug), the mare would be back to normal and pain-free. This had been going on for about eighteen months until the mare went lame and would not on this occasion get better with the usual treatment. It was decision time! I had already told my client that I thought navicular 'disease' unlikely due to the pain appearing to be in only one foot, the feet having relatively good conformation and the acute sudden onset with apparent quick recovery – until this last episode. I should have known better.

We brought the mare in to the clinic and a colleague administered an abaxial nerve block to the affected limb. This makes the posterior part of the foot, including the navicular area, insensitive to pain. Within a few minutes the animal was almost sound. We took a series of X-rays, and it was all too evident after we viewed the second plate that there was something very wrong in the navicular bone. It was easy to see a group of very large holes along the distal (outer) edge of the bone, which were not apparent on the other foot. It just had to be significant.

Since the diagnosis was made the mare has been on a course of Isoxsuprine, which improves the circulation in the foot. This, coupled with corrective shoeing – egg-bar shoes – has had a very good effect and the animal is walking normally again.

This is an atypical case, and just how long the soundness will last is difficult to say, as the lameness may well return after the drug treatment is finished. However, I am hoping that the effects of the Isoxsuprine, occasional pain relief when required, coupled with good shoeing, will keep the animal walking sound for a reasonable length of time. If the condition recurs there are other treatments which can be used, such as neurectomy or cutting the collateral ligaments to the navicular bone. Both these treatments are quite radical and have their advocates in the veterinary profession. Neurectomy is a cheaper option than cutting the ligaments, but it is my opinion that unless the animal is to be retired or to be put in foal the costs involved may not be worthwhile as the patient may never be ridden safely again.

X-ray vision, or short-sightedness?

Many owners with lame horses are prone to phone and request an X-ray for a shoulder or foot, or whatever other part of the limb they suspect is the source of the lameness. I presume this is an attempt to save money by short-circuiting the usual thorough lameness work-up that most vets prefer to do when confronted with a lame horse for which there is no obvious cause, such as an abscess. This involves a series of nerve blocks starting at the foot. The local anaesthetic desensitises the limb from the foot upwards until the lameness disappears. In this way it is possible to pinpoint the probable source of the pain, and the X-ray machine can be directed at that specific point. Using an X-ray alone without nerve blocks may be fruitless unless there is an obvious lesion, such as a swollen knee or hock that is painful to palpate or flex. It is quite possible to X-ray a foot, such as the one I have just described, and see what you suspect is a problem, but if the nerve block is not done, which abolishes the pain, the X-ray will have little value. The two techniques working together are often very necessary to prove a diagnosis. It is short-sighted to attempt to reduce costs by asking for an X-ray alone as this may mislead or delay a proper diagnosis. In cases of non-specific lameness, most equine vets, I'm sure, would not wish to carry out one technique without doing the other. Cost-cutting on lameness can cost you more money in the end.

CHAPTER SEVEN

Teeth

You should look after your horse's teeth as if they were your own. Personally I have a conservation order on all of mine, unlike my mother – bless her – who has had the same false teeth for over sixty years! Horses and ponies are not so fortunate and cannot have adult teeth replaced, so for owners to take care of their horse's teeth makes so much sense. As far as I know sheep are the only animal species to be fitted with false teeth when their natural teeth fall out. It's a curse as well as a blessing for horses that their teeth seem to grow continually throughout their lifetime. In fact, what is actually happening is that as the teeth wear down, the socket from which they come is gradually being filled in, so that the teeth are being pushed out of their sockets. Most horse owners will be unaware that horses and ponies are like rabbits in this respect and teeth problems in rabbits are a major factor in rabbit nutrition, as they are in horse nutrition. The comparison doesn't end there, as rabbits are herbivores, like all equines, and like to graze small amounts frequently; also, they have their main organ of digestion in the caecum.

Ageing horses and ponies by looking at their teeth is a procedure which has been done for many years. When examining an animal for purchase most vets, when there is no documentary evidence of how old the animal is, will look at the teeth and give an opinion as to the animal's age. I always thought it was reasonably possible in a normal mouth to age an animal up to eight years old. After this age it is not possible to be quite so accurate. However, a recent survey among equine vets shook my belief in this accuracy. A group of vets were asked to give an opinion as to the age of a number of horses. The age of each animal was known, but not to the vets. None of the animals was over eight years of age but the results – and it was a group of equine vets who were participating in the trial – were surprising, to say the least. Whilst many were aged correctly, many were not. Some assessments were out by as much as two to three years. It wasn't the vets' fault. They were applying textbook rules to the ageing of teeth, but horses don't always read the books!

When buying a horse or pony the age may really matter. There is a big difference in the horse's value between being eight or eighteen, and the teeth can look very similar to the inexperienced. Whenever possible try and get documentary proof of age, and if this is not available don't try to pin a vet down too much as to precise age. An honest estimate may be the best that can be given.

The oldest pony I knew and treated died aged forty-five and this age was known precisely. Others have been recorded as much older, although these are very rare. Blaine, a veterinary surgeon working in the nineteenth century, looked into the subject of ageing in horses and came to the following conclusions, which still have validity today. He reckoned that five equine years are equivalent to twenty years of human life. So a horse of ten years is equivalent to a man or woman of forty; a horse aged twenty is equivalent to being eighty in human years, which makes my forty-five-year-old pony almost as old as Methuselah!

The adult horse has twelve incisor teeth, which are the biting teeth at the front of the mouth. Six are on the top jaw and six are on the bottom jaw. The animal also has twenty-four molars, which are the grinding teeth; twelve each in both jaws. In addition the adult male has four tushes, or canine teeth, which if present in the mare are very rudimentary. Some individuals also have wolf teeth, which are to be found in front of the upper molars. It is very rare to see wolf teeth in the lower jaw. They are present but rarely come through the gum.

Young horses and ponies have milk teeth, which rarely give trouble and are usually all present by the time the animal is nine months old. Adult teeth replace these temporary teeth, and this process starts in the incisor teeth at the front when the youngster is about two and a half years old. This replacement process goes on until the animal is about four and a half, when all the adult teeth should be present. Very occasionally a milk tooth may become wedged between the adult teeth instead of being dislodged when the adult teeth erupt. If this does happen the horse will have difficulty in eating and may have a foul-smelling breath.

Clients will occasionally worry if they find small lumps along the bottom line of the jawbone. These hard, little pimples along both of the mandibles disappear as the adult molars come through.

If the horse is older than, say, five years and has a hard swelling on one side of the jaw, this will be a time to call for a veterinary opinion. An abscess at the root of a tooth can cause this type of swelling and can result in the horse being in pain and losing condition. An X-ray is usually required to confirm a diagnosis and when this is made the tooth has to be extracted. This means the horse will have to have a general anaesthetic as removing the cheek teeth is a difficult job and will involve the surgeon in question having to use considerable force. There is just no easy way to do the job and it can be costly.

Wolf teeth

The only horse teeth which are comparatively easy to extract are the wolf teeth. These are remnants of teeth which were well developed in the ancient horse breeds which roamed the earth before homo-sapiens put in an appearance.

It was a common belief among horse owners in the Fens of Cambridgeshire, and probably elsewhere as well, that an animal would not thrive properly unless its wolf teeth were removed. More wolf teeth have been removed unnecessarily because of this than bears thinking about. And even today, many vets will remove wolf teeth when it may be totally unnecessary just because they have been requested to do so by a client. A **valid** reason for wolf teeth removal is when the horse is mouthing or playing with the bit, which causes difficulties in controlling the animal when it is being ridden. However, if your horse has wolf teeth and they are not causing a problem, leave them alone. Spending money on having them removed may be a complete waste of time and merely give your animal a very sore mouth for a day or two.

If wolf teeth do have to be removed they come out easily because they have very short roots (unless they belong to Dartmoor ponies, as I know to my cost!). I give the animal a sedative and then loosen the root all around before extracting it with forceps. It used to be the custom

> **More wolf teeth have been removed unnecessarily than bears thinking about.**

for blacksmiths to knock out wolf teeth with a blunt instrument. Thankfully I'm fairly sure that this once common practice has died out completely, as it is now illegal for any lay-person to carry out such 'surgery'.

Jaw, jaw

Overshot jaws are quite common in horses, less so in ponies. This is where the top jaw extends beyond the bottom jaw, and an animal with this type of congenital defect is said to be **parrot-mouthed**. The opposite inherited condition is an undershot jaw, which is quite rare. It is also known as a '**sow mouth**' as it imitates the conformation of a pig's mouth.

Horses and ponies with either type of congenital disorder will manage to graze and eat quite well when they are youngsters. However, after they are a few years old they will be prone to developing hooks in the premolar teeth. This is especially common in parrot-mouthed horses and is the result of a malocclusion of the teeth (this means that the teeth on top and bottom jaws do not meet correctly when the jaw is closed). The top premolar extends beyond the bottom premolar, and as a consequence the front part of the top tooth does not get ground down against its opposite number in the bottom jaw by the chewing action. Eventually a hook is formed which, if left undetected, will grow down and into the gum of the lower jaw causing great discomfort. It is quite simple to check whether your horse has a tendency to be parrot mouthed and if this is the case, a watch must be kept for the development of hooks. Detected early, these hooks can be rasped flat quickly and easily. Left too long it can be a much bigger and more expensive job, as the hooks will need to be sheared off. By the time a parrot-mouthed horse is six years it should have its teeth checked twice a year.

Other congenital disorders of the mouth usually involve cheek teeth (molars) that are missing. When this happens there will be an overgrowth of the tooth, usually in the top jaw, resulting in acute discomfort to the animal as it cannot chew properly, often dropping its food. Dropping food from the mouth for whatever reason is known as **quidding**. A horse that does this regularly needs to have its mouth examined by an expert as soon as possible.

Feeling edgy about the dentist?

As the horse or pony gets older it is very likely to develop sharp edges on the outer edge of the top cheek teeth, which will injure the inside of the cheeks. Sharp edges can also occur on the inner edge of the bottom molars, which can injure the tongue. These edges appear in any normal equine mouth when all the adult teeth are present, due to the upper and lower molars not covering each other entirely. Sharp points must be rasped down on a regular basis, otherwise the animal will not chew properly due to discomfort and it may lose condition and start quidding. It is also possible that it will bolt its food, which could lead to digestive upsets and colic. Sharp teeth, especially the upper premolars, may also be a cause of a horse throwing his head about and fighting the bit.

Many animals need to have their teeth rasped at least once a year, or more often than this if hooks or other sharp edges are present. An experienced person can check for sharp teeth quite readily. The tongue is usually pulled out at the side of the mouth with one hand. This will control the horse to some extent and allow inspection of the cheek teeth on the opposite side. A torch can be useful here. Do not attempt this procedure if you don't know what you are doing, and on no account should you put your fingers up the inside the animal's mouth to check for sharp edges. To get bitten by molar teeth is extremely painful, and I knew a man who lost part of a finger doing just that. It is a much better idea to ask your vet to check the teeth when the animal is having its annual vaccination. In fact, check with the vet to make sure the teeth rasps are carried in the car. If teeth need rasping they can be done at the same time as vaccination and an extra call-out charge will be avoided.

Rasping teeth is usually a fairly easy job if it is done on a regular basis. Most vets will use a mouth gag to hold the jaws open, but this may not always be necessary. Mouth gags are very necessary on some occasions if the animal is prone to biting on the tooth rasp making rasping almost impossible or if the back of the mouth is to be checked properly. Most horses do not mind the procedure too much but there is always the odd rebel. Over the years these troublesome horses have been dealt with by applying a twitch. This instrument consists of a loop of cord attached to a short pole and is applied by twisting the loop tightly around the animal's nose. Modern equivalents – the humane twitch, for example – are usually made of metal and are not so effective. Most horses or ponies go very quiet when twitched – although one can come across the odd exception that cannot be twitched because it makes it totally unmanageable. The twitch works (apparently) by a release of endorphins (morphine-like derivatives) activated by the acupuncture point in the nostrils. Twitching a horse to have its teeth rasped is a cheaper option than sedation, but I have to say I much prefer to sedate the patient by intravenous injection. It gives better, more certain results, is kinder to the animal and avoids the nuisance of the twitch getting

in the way of the rasping procedure.

Over the last few years 'horse
dentists' are increasingly taking
on the role of tooth rasping. Many
of these people do a good job but

> Just as we need regular dental check-ups, so do our equine friends.

they are not true dentists as such, and as lay people are
(strictly speaking) not allowed to remove teeth – this is
an act of veterinary surgery which, under UK law, only
vets are allowed to carry out. I understand that regula-
tions will be put in place to control and license 'horse
dentists' in much the same way as happened to farriers
some years ago. This when it happens will be a very
good thing and will be welcomed by most in the equine
field – not least by the 'dentists' themselves.

Long in the tooth

Old horses are very prone to teeth trouble due to uneven
wear, which can be very difficult to rectify if the animal
has not been checked on a regular basis. Vets in the past
had their own ways of dealing with this type of problem,
which could not be countenanced in these more enlight-
ened times. Even so, over the years I have developed a
huge respect for my veterinary predecessors. The first
document of veterinary medicine is on papyrus and is
very fragmentary, being about four thousand years old.
It seems that the ancient Egyptians had a very good idea
of how to treat various illnesses, based on logic and not
witchcraft. This was carried on through Greek and
Roman times and was then lost during the Dark Ages.
With the advent of the new veterinary schools in France
and then England in the eighteenth century the science
of veterinary medicine once again came to the fore.

I have gathered quite a large collection of antique

veterinary equipment over the years and I have to admit there are one or two instruments that defy identification – I am not sure how they were used or for what purpose. I was browsing through a veterinary instrument catalogue the other day, wondering what to buy – I like new toys – looking for a specific piece of equipment for a patient. The animal needing attention was a thirty-five-year-old pony called Creamy, who had a dental problem. She was dropping more food out of her mouth than she was managing to swallow, and as a consequence was beginning to look very old and thin. A quick glance at her mouth was not very helpful, especially as the old girl was head shy and wouldn't allow me to examine her properly. After a dose of sedative, I put the mouth gag in place and had a good look. There was a large hook on the sixth molar at the back of the bottom jaw. I had difficulty seeing it, but could feel it easily. With the pony very sleepy and the mouth gag in position I could safely put my hand and part of my arm inside her mouth. The hook was long and thick and would make chewing and swallowing very difficult.

Hooks like these are impossible to rasp properly and I needed an instrument to cut off the hook, which was why I was looking through the catalogue. A picture in the brochure of new dental equipment made me realise that I had just the thing I needed in my collection of old veterinary instruments. I had looked at the long, thin rod with a notch at one end before, didn't know for sure what it had been used for, but thought it might have been employed to knock out wolf teeth. I took it from the display cabinet, looked at it again and decided to use it to knock off the offending protuberance. The procedure would not be without some risk. I was concerned that I might crack the molar, but I could not let the animal carry on the way it was. I was also worried that the dislodged tooth particle might fall into the back of the throat and be inhaled into the windpipe.

I went back to see Creamy armed with my ' new' piece of equipment. I followed the usual drill and sedated the old girl with Domosedan. As usual it didn't take very much – although lively, she seemed thinner than ever.

I put the mouth gag into position and once more felt for the offending tooth. It was even longer and thicker than I remembered and I thought once again of the consequences if things went wrong. I couldn't bring myself to attempt to knock the hook off! All too clearly I could see the dangers: if the instrument slipped at the wrong moment, the metal rod might penetrate the soft tissue of the throat or the back of the mouth.

I have this maxim at moments of crisis: 'If you are not sure you are going to do some good, don't do it!'

So I didn't do what I had planned, but I had to do something. I could have referred her to an equine clinic for surgery but the owner wasn't prepared to do this due to the cost and the likelihood of her not surviving a general anaesthetic. To do nothing was not an option. Euthanasia was the only other alternative.

I had with me a pair of long-handled dental forceps, which I thought I might try if all else failed. I reached as far into the mouth as possible and managed to get a grip on the molar, but only just. I had no great hope that I would be able to extract the tooth as equine molars have very long roots, but I had to try. I applied maximum pressure and pulled and twisted. With a crunching noise which will stay with me whenever I get into the dentist chair, it came out. I deposited the offending article into the owner's outstretched hand. I didn't know who was more pleased, him or me, but Creamy couldn't have cared less, as she was still asleep on her feet.

When she did waken there was no doubt that she

could, despite just having had a tooth removed, eat with greater comfort. I hoped that she would soon gain weight and enjoy a more comfortable retirement in her orchard paddock. But it was not to be. After a few more weeks it became apparent that she was not going to put on any more condition, and it was decided to end her life before she became too debilitated.

It was a sad end for her, and very sad for her owners. She had been a very 'hot' little gymkhana pony in her youth, winning trophies far and wide. She had been much loved and pampered when she was active but in retirement, although fed and talked to every day, in other respects she had been somewhat neglected. She should have had had had her teeth checked regularly. Old horses and ponies should be checked at least twice a year whether they are dropping food or not. In this way any defects can be corrected before they become a severe problem. If this had been done then Creamy might have lived much longer, and, who knows, might have outlived my original 'Methuselah'.

Just as we need regular dental check-ups, so do our equine friends. Catch a problem early and it can be put right quickly, easily and without too much cost. Neglect it and it will cost so much more to rectify – it may even be too late for your animal.

CHAPTER EIGHT

Skin Problems – Do They Really Matter?

To the layman, to talk of the skin as an organ may seem somewhat strange. In reality, it is the largest organ in the body and is much more than just an inert covering protecting the inner organs. The skin is a highly complex structure and, even though it is the most accessible organ, its workings are still not completely understood. What we do know is that the skin has to function properly and efficiently for the rest of the body organs to stay healthy.

Its thickness varies from one to five millimetres, depending on which part of the body it covers. Some areas of skin specialise in producing a certain type of hair, e.g. the coarse hair on the mane, tail and poll, and feather as seen on heavy horses. Several coat types have been described. My old anatomy lecturer, Jimmy Speed, said there were five types of coat: a birth coat, a foal coat, a yearling coat, an adult summer coat and an adult winter coat.

The skin itself can become diseased and infected by a variety of bacteria, parasites and fungi; in addition the condition of the skin and coat can be an indicator of internal disorders. An animal that is unwell will lose the bloom or shine from its coat and in some circumstances will retain its winter hair, which is usually a symptom of Cushing's disease.

Testing, testing ...

The vet can readily diagnose many skin diseases by a careful clinical examination, but some conditions need laboratory tests for a proper diagnosis. These can be expensive, but if the vet suggests that tests are necessary don't be put off by the extra costs involved. I have on many occasions been persuaded to forgo tests on economic grounds only to regret it later when the condition has not improved and time has been lost.

One of the easiest tests to carry out is a **skin scraping**. This is where the vet will gently scrape the surface of a lesion with a scalpel blade and the practice laboratory or an external lab will then examine the collected material. This test is extremely useful in the diagnosis of parasitic disease, such as is caused by skin mites like *Chorioptes equi*, which causes immense irritation of the lower limbs of densely feathered horses such as Shires and Clydesdales. Mites such as *Chorioptes* or *Trombiculids* (harvest mite) can only be seen by using a microscope.

Lice and lice eggs are large enough to be seen by the naked eye and these cause irritation and discomfort. The horse or pony that is affected will rub and bite at the skin causing a lot of self-inflicted damage. Lice are usually found in the dense winter coat along the mane and at the base of the tail. They look a bit like specks of dandruff, but if you watch carefully you will see them move! If you are in doubt apply a piece of Sellotape to the skin surface, making sure you pick up some of the suspected pathogens (little blighters!) and take them to your vet for examination.

Lice are either the biting or sucking variety, but it really doesn't matter which type they are as they can be easily and cheaply destroyed by powders or skin washes once the diagnosis is made. Apart from the irritation they cause, sucking lice can result in anaemia by blood sucking and also may be able in this way to transmit other diseases.

If a fungal disease is suspected a **sample of hair** is plucked – not scraped – from the edge of the lesion, so that the roots and shaft of the hairs can be examined by microscopy. If a bacterial infection is to be considered, material has to be obtained from the lesion usually via a **swab**, which is then put into a transport medium and sent to a laboratory for culture and antibiotic sensitivity testing.

The last type of diagnostic skin test is a **biopsy**. Under local anaesthetic a small, round area of skin is removed by a disposable biopsy punch and put into a fixative fluid and then sent to a pathologist who is experienced in looking at equine samples. These samples must always be accompanied by a comprehensive history of the skin disease and multiple samples may have to be taken. This is the most expensive type of skin test and will only be done when there is no other means of reaching a diagnosis.

How well-groomed is your horse?

There is no doubt that an owner or groom has a vital role to play in the prevention of skin disease in the stabled horse. This role doesn't cost any money but it can be hard work and time-consuming. It is called grooming.

Grooming promotes a healthy skin by stimulating the circulation and glands. It opens the skin pores and removes dirt, skin debris and sweat. A stabled horse should be groomed daily.

A horse at grass that is not being ridden should not be groomed (for reasons given below) but must be checked daily and have its feet picked out every day. Rolling is a self-grooming process for the horse at pasture, and most

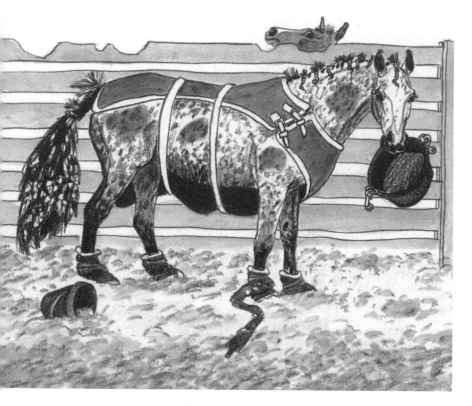

The show-groom's nightmare.

horses in a group will engage in mutual grooming sessions.

It is better not to shampoo a horse too often, unless otherwise advised by your vet, as this may disturb the underlying grease, which acts as weatherproofing. In cold weather if an animal has to be washed, make sure it is dried thoroughly afterwards and protected from the cold. Very muddy horses should have their legs washed down with water and then dried well with

> **Don't use a dandy brush to clean the mud from the legs as this can damage the skin surface and allow bacteria or spores to penetrate the epidermis.**

towels or bandages. Don't use a dandy brush to clean the mud from the legs as this can damage the skin surface and allow bacteria or spores to penetrate the epidermis. If an animal has been sweating heavily it may be washed down all over without harm, but the excess water should be removed with a sweat-scraper. If it is cold or windy towel dry the back and loins to avoid chills. If this is not possible an alternative is to protect the horse with a sweat sheet and walk the animal until it is dry.

Dermatophilosis – a.k.a. mud fever, greasy heel, rain scald, etc.

One of the many problems vet students and new graduates have to deal with is diseases which have different names depending on who they are talking to and where they are in the country.

Dermatophilosis is one of these diseases. It can be, and has been, called streptothricosis, mycotic dermatitis, rain scald, mud fever, greasy heel – and these are just a few of the most used names. All these conditions have one thing in common. A fungal organism, an actinomycete, called *Dermatophilus congolensis* causes them all, and they are all different manifestations of the same disease. It is a disease, which is just as commonly found in tropical climates as in temperate ones. The common factor is rain, especially heavily driving rain and mud, which allows the spore stage of the infection to penetrate the skin.

As I have already mentioned, the depth of the skin varies from site to site and also to some extent from breed to breed. For example, the skin on the chest wall is very different from the skin on the legs, just as the skin of a Shetland is quite different in structure to that of, say, a Shire. Knowing this helps to explain why rain scald on an animal's back will look quite different from mud fever on a leg, although it is the same disease condition. Similarly it will also explain why some breeds are more prone to some skin infections than others. Thoroughbreds are notoriously thin-skinned and liable to skin infection, and ponies are more likely to suffer from sweet itch than horses.

Fortunately, this skin disease – dermatophilus – is relatively easy to diagnose by an experienced equine vet, but hair plucks and skin scrapings will readily prove a diagnosis.

Clinical signs of the disease vary according to the severity of the infection. In the winter months, especially when the weather has been very wet but mild, mud fever and rain scald can be very bad.

When an animal has **rain scald**, 'paint brush' tufts of hair will be very apparent, particularly over the body where it is liable to be most wet: the back, the shoulders and the flanks. Saucer-shaped scabs appear with moist purulent material under the scabs. If the condition is long-standing, this purulent material can dry out but leaves the skin underneath pink and wet.

Where **mud fever** is present on the legs, the lesions look crusty and yellow. The skin underneath the crusts will be dry, cracked and very sore. The legs will also become swollen and the animal may well be lame. If left untreated too long the legs could become permanently thickened. The only redeeming feature of a dermatophilus infection is that it is not itchy.

> **If mud fever is left untreated too long the legs could become permanently thickened.**

Horses and ponies that are kept out all the time in the winter without protection are very susceptible, and if any are in poor condition the infection will really catch hold. I examined two emaciated yearlings last winter on behalf of the RSPCA and both had the most severe rain scald I have ever seen, which I am sure was made much worse by the animals' very poor general condition. Both horses were covered with a dense mattress of purulent, dry, scabby material, which covered the entire chest and the back areas. They looked terrible and I am sure must have been very miserable. The owners were successfully prosecuted.

Treatment of the disease is relatively straightforward and there is much the owner can do in concert with the vet, which will save money. As the major cause is prolonged exposure to moisture and poor hygiene then the first step should be to house the patient. Long hair should be clipped off and the affected areas washed with an antiseptic wash such as Hibiscrub or Povidone. The affected area should then be dressed with an antiseptic cream, and severe infections will require either daily injections of antibiotic or antibacterial treatment given in the feed or by oral paste. This treatment must be under the care and supervision of your vet.

Prevention is always better than cure. Practise good husbandry – it will save you lots of money!

Always provide a field shelter in wet weather, especially if the animal is not protected by a New Zealand rug. On returning from a hack, to prevent mud fever, wash the legs down with water and dry them thoroughly afterwards. I believe that this is more effective than allowing the skin and hair to dry and then brushing clean, but you must ensure the skin and hair is dry as soon as possible after washing.

These are simple measures, which work well. If you still find your animal has a skin problem of the above nature, get treatment as soon as possible as the condition will only get worse and cost you more in the end.

Ringworm

Ringworm is an unfortunate name for this disease as it has nothing to do with worms; it is caused by a type of fungal infection. The name can still strike dread and despondency into owners of riding schools and livery yards, or wherever numbers of horses are congregated.

The last outbreak I dealt with was in a riding school, which catered for, among others, disabled riders and quite young children. The owner was very concerned about the cost of eradicating the disease but was also acutely aware that the infection could be passed on to her human clients. The disease itself does not cause serious illness, but it is unsightly and very contagious, and the spores, which carry the infection, are difficult to eradicate from a building. In fact, spores can survive for years in the crevices of buildings, on wooden fences and, of course, in any vehicle used for transporting animals. The infection is also spread very rapidly if communal tack or grooming equipment becomes infected. Young animals and children are especially at risk, and it is very common to find the disease in yearlings that have just come through a sale-ring. The incubation period is about two weeks.

Ringworm in Britain is caused by one of two pathogenic fungi. One is trichophyton, which commonly infects cattle, and the other is microsporum, which is more common in dogs and cats. In the outbreak in the riding school, the cause was identified as microsporum, and the stable cats and dogs came under suspicion straightaway.

> Ringworm spores can survive for years, in the crevices of buildings, on wooden fences, etc.

The appearance of the disease varies quite a lot but the lesions are seen typically around the areas which come into contact with rugs, tack or even riding boots. Where there is mild rubbing to the surface of the skin, this breaks the surface integrity and can allow the fungal infection to gain a hold. The disease then becomes established. The early signs on the skin are of more or less circular areas about one to two centimetres in diameter with the hairs being raised and tufted above the scabs. Once any purulent material has dried off and the scab comes away, it leaves an area with a dry, scaly appearance. In foals it is not uncommon for the infected areas to be much larger and for the lesions to be covered with a thick grey scale.

Most veterinary surgeons are able to diagnose ringworm very readily but some cases may be open to doubt. It is also not possible to identify which type of fungal infection is involved without resorting to laboratory testing. Hair samples can be examined under a microscope, which will usually reveal the fungal spores along the hair follicle giving it a sheathed appearance.

Microsporum infection, if viewed in the dark, will give off a characteristic green glow if ultraviolet light is shone on the sample. If there is still doubt about the result, the lab will culture the sample to identify the fungus, but this can take up to two weeks.

It is not usually realised that in the summer many ringworm infections will get better if the animal is kept outside, but it will take at least to two to three months. This is because the action of the ultraviolet rays from the sun coupled with the animal's natural immunity will get rid of the infection.

This being the case, why do we bother to treat the infection in the first place?

Firstly because it is unsightly and causes irritation and inflammation to the affected animal. It also affects people, especially children and teenagers. However, the main reason for treating the infection is to minimise spread of what is a very contagious organism in the environment, and to stop the infection causing havoc to other horses and other animals.

If only one animal is infected it should be isolated, the affected area clipped and the lesion dressed with an antifungal preparation. Mycophyt (made by Intervet) is a very effective drug for this purpose and can be sprayed or sponged onto the infected area every four to five days. It is very safe and can be used in pregnant animals, as it is not absorbed through the skin.

Antimycotic agents can also be given by mouth in the feed. Griseofulvin is the active principal involved and it is supplied under a variety of trade names. It is very effective but more expensive than other ringworm treatments. It will cost about the price of a tank full of petrol to treat one horse for seven days, which is the normal course that is required.

The drug must be used with extreme caution, as it must not be given to pregnant mares. Women of child-bearing age, even if they are not pregnant, should avoid contact with the drug as it can damage foetuses and result in terrible deformities in the newborn.

Other preparations such as iodine or copper sprays can be bought in tack shops, which can have some value in treatment, but I recommend that you stick to licensed products, which are only obtainable through your vet.

When treating ringworm you should always wear gloves, although you will find many vets don't bother (especially the older, more gnarled variety) as they have long since become immune to the disease.

You should keep all tack and grooming equipment specifically for one horse to avoid or limit the spread of infection. Tack and equipment from an infected animal should be thoroughly cleaned with soap and water and can be immersed or sprayed with an antifungal agent such as Mycophyt. Isolate the individual concerned if possible, avoid contact with other horses and treat the infection just as soon as possible.

If it is at all possible, treat all surfaces, including stable surfaces and fittings, to kill off the fungal spores. This can be done with a pressure hose, and formalin can be used as well. However, formalin has to be used with great care as it can be irritating to the eyes (it makes me cough!). Mycophyt can also be used very safely for this purpose.

Fencing and all wooden surfaces can be given a coating with creosote, which not only preserves the wood, but also kills fungal spores. Horses and ponies should not be put back into stables that have been freshly treated with creosote as this might cause skin and eye irritations. A few days should be allowed to lapse to allow the creosote smell to diminish and the woodwork to dry out.

Simple control measures such as these are inexpensive but can do much to reduce the anguish and often hysteria, which often is the result of a diagnosis of ringworm. Act promptly and the disease will be under control and gone much quicker than might otherwise happen if you delay.

Sweet itch - not so sweet

The correct scientific name for sweet itch is allergic arthropod dermatitis, but like most scientific labels by the time you have learned it some one will have changed it to something else even more obscure. It may be called by other local names such as **summer eczema** or **Queensland itch**, but sweet itch describes the condition very well.

It is an allergic skin disorder, which can occur in any age of animal over a year old but is most common in ponies. It is often seen in horses – hacks and hunters – but I have never seen it in a heavy horse. It is also suggested that it is more rare in Thoroughbreds.

In Britain the disease is seasonal, mostly from April to October, and is due to the affected animal being hypersensitive to the biting midge (Culicoides).

It is the female of the species that causes the trouble as it only is the blood-sucker (and as a mere man that is the only sexist comment I am going to make!).

The signs of the condition are fairly self evident and are the result of an intense itch, making the animal rub its mane and rub and bite at the base of the tail. This causes a loss of hair and an oozing of serum from the skin, which initially gives the skin a wet look. This soon, however, dries out to leave a crusty appearance, and chronic cases will have areas of dry, thickened, ridged skin. The mane and tail can look terrible due to hairs being lost and broken. I have known a few ponies to be so badly affected that they were unworkable.

Over the years many different treatments have been tried. Benzyl benzoate, either neat or in liquid paraffin, has been used topically, but I have never thought it to be especially effective. Much more useful is the range of synthetic pyrethrin repellents (such as Switch) which are applied along the back of the animal every six days. Steroid cream applied topically will give temporary relief, but this is only treating the symptoms and not the cause. This also true of steroid injections, which will give relief from the itching, but must be treated with great caution by your vet as steroids can bring on an attack of laminitis, especially in overweight ponies.

Midges bite mostly at dawn and dusk or when the weather is very hot and humid. Control is based on keeping the susceptible animals housed between dawn and ten in the morning and from four in the afternoon until dark. Anti-midge screens in the stable may help to prevent midge access, and a Vapona strip may knock out any that penetrate the screen. If you can't stable the animal please keep it away from fields with trees, hedges and ponds, which is where the midges are to be found.

Sweet itch is a distressing condition for all concerned, sometimes even the vet. A few years ago I vetted a pony – it was April/ May time – for purchase and passed it as sound for the purposes for which it was required. It left its bare open fenland field for pastures new and within weeks the new owner was on the phone to complain that the pony had sweet itch and why did I not see the problem when I vetted it for her?

She took a lot of convincing that the skin was in good condition at the time of purchase and that I, let alone anyone else, had no knowledge that the pony was allergic to midge bites. Although it was some distance away, I went to see it and whilst I could see no midges on the animal – as you can sometimes – the evidence of the skin allergy was all too apparent. However, the problem lay with the field the pony now occupied. It was beautifully sheltered on all sides with a thick hedge, and it had a stream running through one side. Idyllic, you might think, but only for the midges – not for the patient. If asked, I suspect the pony would have much preferred to be back in its windswept fen field, where midges seldom dare to venture out.

It was not possible to stable the pony, so I suggested a change of pasture to a more open field and advised the use of a pour-on midge repellent. I never saw the pony again but I was informed that the problem was kept within manageable levels, though not completely cured.

Simple, easy and cheap solutions should keep your pony comfortable and avoid the necessity of expensive veterinary treatments.

Lumps and bumps

Lumps and bumps on the skin can be alarming for many owners. Some are fairly innocuous but can sometimes be a nuisance. **Saddle sores** and **girth galls** come into this category and are preventable by checking the saddle area frequently for early evidence of unnatural pressure, heat or loss of hair and swelling. Saddles should be clean and checked regularly for uneven wear and to make sure they fit properly. If sores do happen and become infected by neglect they should be cleaned with a mild antiseptic solution and treated with an antibiotic cream supplied by your vet. Chronic swellings around the withers have to be carefully protected to stop them becoming larger, and I find that talcum powder applied profusely under any saddle padding can be useful.

Urticarial plaques are large raised nodules some the size of fifty pence pieces, which come up very quickly all over the body. They are caused by **allergic reactions** to insect bites, such as from the common house-fly, but can also be the result of an allergic reaction to substances in the feed or even to an injection. These plaques, or nodules, may go down as quickly as they appeared, but if the animal is distressed, it may require veterinary attention.

Ear plaques are white or grey raised areas in the inner surface of the ear. No one is really sure what causes this condition but if your horse develops them, do not worry. Treatment is unavailing and unnecessary and you need not trouble your vet.

Acne, similar to teenage acne, is the result of the skin getting infected with the bacteria *Staphylococcus epidermis.* Small pustules can appear anywhere on the skin but are most common in the saddle area. Like for any teenager, the treatment for mild cases is antiseptic skin-washes with Hibiscrub or iodine-based washes

> **Horses with mild cases of sunburn can be protected by high-factor sun block. Severe cases have to be stabled.**

(Povidone) and if the condition is severe your vet may have to prescribe topical or systemic antibiotics. There is little doubt that acne can often be the result of poor hygiene and lack of grooming. It is most often seen during mild, wet winters.

In the summer months, though, it is not uncommon to see **sunburned** horses. Light-skinned horses can be badly burned on non-pigmented areas, such as the muzzle and tips of the ears. Ingestion of some plants such as St Johns Wort can make the animal more sensitive to the effects of the sun. Severe cases have to be stabled; mild cases will be protected by high-factor sun block applied frequently.

Some systemic diseases can be readily diagnosed by the effect the condition has on the animal's skin. **Purpura haemorrhagica** is a case in point. This illness occurs after a bacterial infection such as strangles and is the result of an immunological reaction. Capillaries and blood vessels are damaged, which results in fluid leakage into the subcutaneous tissues. The skin seems to ooze serum and the legs and under the belly fill with fluid. It is obvious to all that the animal is severely ill. The prospects for recovery from this condition are very guarded.

If you have a pony or horse with these symptoms get help as soon as possible as the quicker treatment is given, the better.

Warts an' all

Skin tumours cannot be prevented by good management or by wrapping your animal in cotton wool. The veterinary profession has no means as yet to prevent the occurrence of **warts**, **sarcoids**, or **melanoma**, which are the most common forms of skin cancer in the horse.

I was thinking about this, trying to take my mind off my immediate position as I crouched under the belly of a 16hh bay gelding, which was swaying just a little on its hind legs. I was about to place on the animal's skin the modern equivalent of a hot iron – a diathermy instrument. If the animal fell over, I was going to be crushed, and if it was going to kick – well it didn't bear thinking about. If the health and safety inspector could see me now, I thought, without even a hard hat for protection.

The reason for my apparent vulnerability was an operation I was about to carry out for the removal of a sarcoid from the animal's groin. Sarcoids, for some reason unknown to me, always seem to occur in the most inaccessible places, or perhaps I only remember the difficult cases.

Sarcoids are skin tumours, and are the most common type of skin cancer found in the horse, donkey or mule. They are caused by a virus infection and are different in appearance and size to warts. Warts are smaller and mostly disappear within a few months, especially if the animal is young.

Like warts, sarcoids are benign tumours, meaning they do not metastasise (spread) to the rest of the body, but they do tend to recur after surgical removal.

They can occur anywhere on the body, but the head, neck, lower chest and belly and, of course, the groin are the normal areas of involvement. They tend to be classified by appearance and into four different types.

The verrucose type are a bit like warts but bigger,

usually up to 6cm in diameter and often pedunculated (with a narrow neck).

Fibroplastic sarcoids are small, firm and fibrous and often seen around the eyes. Verrucose and fibroplastic sarcoids can exist together and often become ulcerated and infected.

Nodular sarcoids, the last type, can extend over quite a large area with associated hair loss and small skin nodules. Although all types of sarcoid can come back after removal, nodular sarcoids can be the most difficult to treat as they can spread over quite a large area before veterinary assistance is requested.

Crouched as I was under my patient I was looking at what I considered to be a verrucose sarcoid, fairly small – just over a fifty pence piece in size – with no evidence of any spread elsewhere.

I had sedated the animal with Domosedan, which is a very powerful drug but does cause the patient to sway a bit on the hind legs. I have only ever had one horse lie down under the influence of the drug, and I hoped this horse wasn't about to do the same.

I managed to infiltrate the area around the tumour with local anaesthetic without a problem and I was now ready for the operation. I was going to use diathermy to remove the lump. The equipment is a hand-held device, which at the touch of the trigger puts a current through the blade, making it red-hot. The blade cuts and burns at the same time, which is very useful as the tumour comes away and there is no bleeding.

This particular sarcoid was no exception to the rule and was removed without incident. I did not

Don't wait to see if a lump is going to get any bigger before asking for professional advice. You may be endangering your horse.

stitch the skin afterwards as I have found from bitter experience that by using a traditional scalpel and suturing the skin, the sarcoid is much more likely to grow again.

Although diathermy is my favoured method of removing sarcoids I much prefer to treat them before they get too big by injecting a chemo-therapeutic drug into the tumour. This causes the cancer to regress and disappear and can be much less stressful to the horse. It is also much cheaper for the client, but you have to treat early to make this method feasible.

Other methods for treating sarcoids include cryosurgery, which involves the use of liquid nitrogen to freeze the tumour, or the insertion of radio-active needles.

This last method can be useful if the sarcoid is very close, as some are, to the eye, but most practices would have to refer patients to specialist practices for this type of treatment, and the use of the new chemo-therapeutic drug called cisplatin may make the needle treatment redundant. Cisplatin is a very toxic drug, which must be used with extreme care. You will find that vets using this treatment will wear gloves and eye protection.

Melanomas are extremely malignant tumours found around the anal area in old grey horses. If detected early, surgical removal is possible, but many are ignored and the usual scenario is that the animal eventually has colic due to spread of the tumour and the outcome is invariably fatal.

If you find an unexplained lump on your horse, please seek advice early. It may well be nothing to worry about, but waiting to see if it is going to get any bigger before asking for professional advice may endanger your horse and may make any treatment or surgery much more expensive.

Cushing's disease

Cushing's disease occurs in older horses and ponies and is the result of a usually benign cancer of the pituitary gland in the brain. This gland secretes hormones, which control all the other endocrine glands in the body and therefore the general body metabolism. The gland enlarges and produces high doses of hormones, which affect the adrenal glands, which are near the kidneys. This results in an over-production of cortisone. The most obvious sign of the disease is to be seen in the spring when the animal looks like a 'woolly bear' as it just refuses to shed its winter coat. Eventually the patient will become quite ill and be very prone to laminitis. Cushing's disease is quite easy to diagnose because of the way the animal looks, although the illness needs to be confirmed by blood sample. Treatment is now much improved and offers some hope to owners who may wish to choose that option. Cushing's disease cannot be prevented by any known means but the effects can be much mitigated by early treatment.

CHAPTER NINE

Exercise-Induced Problems

Many horses are highly specialised, finely tuned athletes and as such are very prone to accident or injury. Racehorses and those competing in long-distance events come most readily to mind. But most horses and ponies, unless they are very young or pensioned off, are liable to injury when they are at work, be it ever so humble as a gentle hack or pulling a cart. Many injuries can be avoided, as explained already, by making sure the feet are in good condition, properly and regularly shod. Horses are like human athletes: before being asked to work hard, they must be given time to warm up. Bringing a horse out of the stable and putting it into a gallop straight away is just asking for trouble! You would not expect a football player to do it, nor should you expect it of a horse or pony.

Fast work on a hard surface such as roadway, or jumping on hard ground can, if it is sustained, cause the animal bruising to the feet, concussion laminitis, sore shin-bones and splints. The result of thoughtless riding may be an animal off work for weeks before soreness as the result of bruising goes away.

All tied up?

One of the most difficult exercise-related conditions to contend with is **azoturia**. This disease has been called by many names, such as **rhabdomyolosis, tying up, setfast** or **Monday morning disease**, and is seen when an animal (and it is usually a horse) develops muscle stiffness and pain while it is being exercised. The symptoms will vary from mild hind-leg stiffness, to sweating heavily as the result of severe pain, and even to total reluctance to move. Animals with the severe form of the disease will pass very dark-coloured urine due to the release of myoglobin from damaged muscles. Milder cases will not show this symptom but a blood test will rapidly confirm a clinical diagnosis. Severely ill animals have been known to become recumbent and die.

On a superficial level the cause of the condition has been known for many years. It typically occurs in a high-performance animal, which is being fed a concentrate ration rich in carbohydrate when the horse is not being exercised. It will have been working hard, and then has a day off but the ration is not reduced, and when the horse returns to work the symptoms appear. This bad management causes a breakdown of the muscle cells and the release of myoglobin due to the build up of lactic acid in the muscles.

Unfortunately this cannot be the complete picture as some horses I know have recurrent attacks despite the greatest care being taken with their feeding regime. It is thought that such animals may have electrolyte imbalances. The most important electrolytes in the body are sodium, potassium, chloride, magnesium and calcium and these must be in the correct balance. This balance can only be checked properly by looking at combined urine and blood samples.

If you suspect your horse might have the illness, don't hesitate to get the vet. Continuing to work the animal believing it might work off a 'cramp attack' may make the condition much worse. If it happens a distance from home, **transport it back.** If the animal is severely affected a delay could mean that the animal might go down and be unable to rise again – and may die. Until professional help arrives cut out all hard feed and give access to hay and water only. The vet will give pain-relief, usually into the vein, and if the horse is very distressed it may be necessary to sedate the patient as well.

Prevention is vital, and being careful with feeding and management will prevent all but the most difficult cases. If the horse has a day off, the concentrate ration should be much reduced or even in some cases not given at all. Do not feed bran instead, as bran can cause an imbalance between phosphate and calcium in the horse. A bran mash given once a week is fine for a normal animal, but if the horse is prone to azoturia do not feed it at all.

It is also important to allow the animal time to **warm up before any strenuous work.**

If your animal has a chronic problem your vet may identify an electrolyte imbalance, which will have to be put right. On a simple level this may involve adding salt to the diet and trying to ensure that after a break from strenuous exercise the horse has a drink of an electrolyte solution, which will replace vital minerals lost with sweating. You can refute the old saying about 'taking a horse to water' by training it to have drink when instructed. This is especially important for animals on long-distance rides.

Feed a balanced diet as advised by a nutritionist. I am constantly amazed that so many horse owners mix different rations from different sources with very little idea of what they could be doing to their horse. This can be disastrous. Please consult your vet or a qualified nutritionist. Feed companies employ such people to give advice and although that advice may be slanted towards

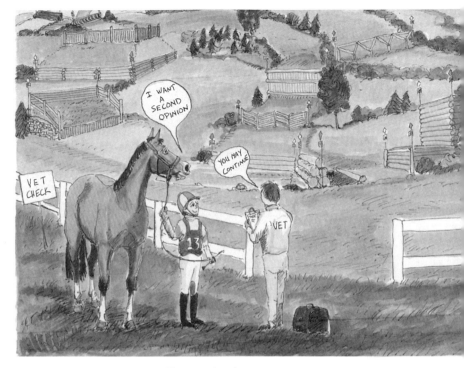

The vet check.

their company products it nonetheless will be better in most instances than a hit-or-miss approach.

Hot, hot, hot

Horses and ponies competing when the weather is hot are very liable to get overheated and could suffer from heat stress. The normal temperature for a horse is 100.5°F (37–38°C). A temperature above 104°F (40°C) is potentially serious and the animal needs to be cooled down as soon as possible. The Animal Health Trust at Newmarket have researched the subject very fully and have devised a cooling technique, which is very safe and allows the animal to recover, perform better and does not cause tying up or azoturia, which has been suggested in the past.

Cooling down method
Cold water is applied liberally to all parts of the body including the quarters, as the large muscles there get particularly hot. Use a sponge and large buckets of cold water, and ice if you can get it. Do this for up to thirty seconds and then walk the animal for thirty seconds and repeat the water applications. It is important to have this walking sequence between the cold-water applications as this promotes skin blood-flow and the movement of air aids evaporation. If it is possible, conduct both the cooling and walking in the shade. Continue this treatment until the horse's temperature has returned to normal or it starts to shiver. At the same time the breathing rate should be much reduced and no more than thirty breaths to the minute. Allowing the horse a small drink (half a bucket) at natural intervals, for example between rounds if it is a show jumper, will help stop the onset of overheating.

A bloody nose?

Nosebleeds, or epistaxis, which is the correct technical name for the condition, occur most often with exercise and are surprisingly common in horses. Most clients are concerned when their horse has a nasal haemorrhage. Sometimes this is justified and sometimes not, but all cases should be investigated.

A proper investigation starts with taking a history and this is usually done – at least initially – over the telephone. My latest case began in this way. The client informed me that she was worried about a nosebleed in her Thoroughbred mare, which had occurred on at least three occasions over the last month. This time it was not associated with exercise and the animal did not have a cough. All this information was very helpful as already I was building up a picture of the likeliest possibilities. However, the only way to determine exactly what was going on was to give the animal a complete clinical examination. In addition, it would be necessary to pass a flexible endoscope up the nostril into the back of the throat and then down the windpipe to examine the lungs. An endoscope is a fibre-optic tube, which allows the clinician to visualise and examine potential lesions deep inside the animal's chest. It is done while the animal is conscious but usually sedated, and the technique will probably cost no more than one hundred pounds which, considering the endoscope can cost up to five thousand pounds to buy, is good value for money.

Bilateral nosebleeds (both nostrils at the same time) are potentially the most alarming and possibly life-threatening, which is why they should never be ignored. The common cause of these nosebleeds is haemorrhage from the lungs at fast exercise. This is often called in lay terms 'bursting a blood vessel'. If the animal is bleeding from the lung tissue, the endoscope will show evidence of blood in the windpipe. Samples of mucus can also be taken, which will help determine if there is disease present in the lung tissue.

The cause of lung bleeding is not really understood but thought to be due to mechanical stress to lung tissue. At a gallop, the animal is breathing very forcefully which can cause delicate air cells to rupture. This can happen in normal lungs but if the horse has a lung condition such as chronic obstructive pulmonary disease (COPD) or a bacterial or viral lung infection this will make the bleeding more likely to occur. In those cases caused by lung disease, treating the underlying condition will go a long way to stopping a recurrence of the haemorrhage.

Fungal infections of the guttural pouch, which are two structures at the back of the throat, can cause bilateral bleeding. This is potentially a very serious disease and the bleeding is often not associated with exercise. In addition to haemorrhage, there is usually a chronic purulent nasal discharge. If this type of bleeding is ignored, the consequences could be fatal as a fungal infection in the guttural pouch can cause ulceration of the carotid artery. The haemorrhage from there can be sudden, massive and fatal. I have seen one horse die like this in front of my eyes. There was nothing that I or anyone else could do, and it was a truly awful sight.

An endoscope examination will check both pouches for signs of infection, and if the animal is at risk of bleeding profusely, then surgery may be required. If the condition is not too severe, flushing the pouches with antibiotic or anti-fungal preparations via an indwelling catheter may cure the infection

As I started my examination on this particular patient, I was reasonably sure from the history that I was unlikely to encounter a major problem, but you can never be too sure. The mare looked in good order and, using a stethoscope, I examined her chest and there was no evidence of lung disease. Palpation of the throat failed to make her cough, which is a symptom of even mild COPD. There were no signs of a nasal discharge, even from the one nostril which had bled.

> **Never ignore a nosebleed; it might prove fatal for the horse the next time.**

With the patient sedated I managed to visualise all the way up the nose, into the throat and down the windpipe. All with negative results!

There did seem to be some

signs of scar tissue halfway up the nasal septum, which may have been the origin of the bleeding, but it was difficult to be sure. In this case I was able to reassure my client that the mare was not going to have a massive haemorrhage and she could carry on riding her horse. Negative findings from a clinician's point of view are difficult, as it then becomes impossible to say whether the condition will recur. If the bleeding persisted, I wanted to examine the horse again as soon as possible after a bleed, even a minor one, as it then might be possible to pinpoint the source of the haemorrhage. Never ignore a nosebleed; it might prove fatal for the horse the next time.

Splints and broken bones

I mentioned splints at the beginning of the chapter, which can be the result of concussion on hard ground. They can also be the result of poor foot balance causing the animal to have an uneven action, which results in the tearing of the interosseous ligament, which attaches the splint bone to the cannon bone. Other causes, equally preventable, are a poor diet resulting in mineral imbalances (don't feed bran as a routine to young horses), or trauma, such as a self-inflicted kick due to faulty action or conformation, or, unpreventable, a kick from another horse. The result is a hard, bony swelling on the side of the horse's leg which, although unsightly, causes very little trouble apart from some initial lameness.

In the early stages the animal is lame due to pain and soft tissue swelling, but this tissue swelling is replaced quite quickly by calcification and new bone is produced beneath the membrane that lines the bone. This results in a firm union between the splint and cannon bones and at this stage all lameness will be gone.

The most important treatment for a splint is the cheapest of all – complete rest. This means at least six weeks off work, preferably box rest, and sometimes longer if necessary. If you put the animal back to work too soon, even if there are no signs of pain or lameness, you may aggravate the problem and enlarge the splint still further. If a splint is diagnosed very early it can be useful to use cold applications, such as hosing or cold packs to reduce the soft tissue swelling. If the condition is diagnosed later, anti-inflammatory drugs may be given by mouth or dimethyl sulphoxide (DMSO) applied to the affected area.

I am often asked if it is possible to surgically remove large splints for cosmetic reasons. It is possible, but I don't recommend doing it, as the outcome can't be guaranteed. Surgery may remove a splint but the very act may stimulate further bone development and the end result may be not much better than the original defect. Surgery would be indicated if the splint is badly placed and is interfering with the horse's action.

Most splints conform to the pattern as described but as with most things in veterinary medicine, now and again they don't.

A recent case involved a horse, which was slightly lame with a moderate swelling over the splint area on the left hind leg. I thought almost certainly the animal had been kicked and I prescribed painkillers and some antibiotics as the skin was cut slightly.

> **The most important treatment for a splint is the cheapest of all – complete rest.**

I rechecked after three days. In the box the patient showed no signs of discomfort, but as the swelling had not reduced, I advised the owner, just to be on

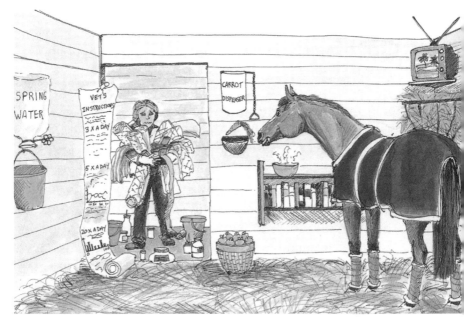

Box rest.

the safe side, to have the leg X-rayed. I went back the next day and was most surprised to find the splint bone had been fractured in three places.

Most of the time with this type of fracture, strict box rest for at least six weeks is required followed by very restricted exercise for two to three months. Most of these fractures heal spontaneously and persistent lameness is unusual.

If you attempt to start exercise too soon you will only delay the animal's recovery and possibly make the splint look even bigger. I know this too well from another case, which was referred to a specialist practice in Newmarket due to persistent lameness resulting from a splint. A fragment of splint bone was removed, which seemed to be the cause of the problem. However, the owner, despite being told very carefully what she should and should not do with her horse chose to ignore the advice after a month and turned him out in a paddock. He romped around the field, as all young animals do, and completely undid all the good work that had been done.

It took nine more months of care and attention before he was sound again. The only consolation for all concerned was that unlike a lot of horses with a broken leg, which technically he had, he at least, in the end, made a good recovery. It was also good to remember that not all horses with broken legs have to be put down.

Unfortunately fractures to the major bones in horses are still very common, always dramatic and, even in these modern times, liable to end with the death of the horse. It is vital that if you suspect your animal may have sustained a major fracture while out exercising to stop and get off immediately and summon professional help. The only excuse for moving at all is if the animal is on a road and may be at further risk from traffic. This is true as well if the horse has been hit by a vehicle and badly hurt. Don't move it until help arrives, unless it is really at risk of another collision.

The reason behind this piece of advice is that if a bone is fractured, there is a much better chance of surgical repair if the bony fragments are kept immobile, less soft tissue damage will occur and the horse will be in less pain if not moved. The vet has to make an on-the-spot assessment and if a possible fracture is confirmed, the leg has to be immobilised by effective emergency splinting which should stop the fracture becoming worse before the animal is moved. There will be occasions where it is obvious to the vet that nothing can be done and the horse may have to be put down there and then to avoid further suffering.

The last major episode of this type in which I was involved was fairly typical.

The instructions over the radio-telephone were quite

clear. 'Take the first turn on the left after the pub. Follow the road until you can go no further. Park the car and walk along the tow-path beside the river and you should come across the horse with the broken leg within a few hundred yards.'

Messages like this are part and parcel of practice life (fortunately not too frequent) and never fail to quicken the pulse. Your mind goes into overdrive as you think ahead of the possible problems you will encounter and how best to deal with them. No matter how many emergency situations you encounter, no two are the same and an individual solution has to be reached for each different case.

The directions were perfect, and I arrived at the scene to find a colleague had got there before me. The horse was a quiet bay gelding who showed no signs of pain apart from in its hind leg, which was resting with a toe pointed to the ground. The owner had been very sensible and explained the horse had stumbled when someone had jumped off a boat, which was moored nearby. She, the owner, had realised something was badly wrong immediately and with great presence of mind had not tried to move the animal in any way. The examination of the limb was straightforward and it was all too apparent from crepitus (or grating) over the area that the pastern bone or first phalanx was fractured.

This type of fracture is unfortunately not uncommon and used to be known as a split pastern. It is seen most frequently in the front legs of racehorses and hunters. This case was a hind leg, which made it a little more unusual.

Often the fracture is a simple longitudinal or trans-verse break with very little displacement. I feared this was not the case with this patient due to the amount of grating I could feel. We had to move the horse. The tow-path was narrow with no prospect of getting a horsebox near the patient. While I administered an intravenous pain-killing injection, my colleague organised a very effective splint out of some lightweight wooden planking, lots of cotton wool and elasticated bandages.

When the foot was totally immobilised, the horse was easily persuaded to walk on three legs to the end of the path and onto a low-loading trailer. A padded partition and bales of straw were put in place, which allowed it to balance and compensate for not being able to use its broken leg.

The driver was told to drive very steadily and to avoid any sudden breaking or acceleration. It's not possible to consider the treatment options for this type of fracture without X-rays. These are simple enough to do, as any reasonable portable machine will give good results. However, in this case, the only hope of possibly repairing the leg was to send the patient to Newmarket to a veterinary orthopaedic surgeon. There was just a chance that this treatment would be successful.

The patient had a good journey without obvious problems. The fractured leg was still effectively immobilised, which was vital if a repair was to be attempted. Sadly, in this case the bone was broken into nine different pieces. There was no hope of it being repaired by orthopaedic screws. Even if the bones could have been screwed together to allow healing, the joint was compromised. This meant that any weightbearing on the leg would have forced the fragments apart and severe arthritis would be the outcome. There was no other way, despite every one's best efforts, but to put the animal down to avoid further suffering, and this was done without delay. This was very sad as the previous year, a horse in similar circumstances sustained a fracture of the same bone caused by its foot slipping off a kerb. In this case the bone was broken in only one place and was successfully repaired.

I am quite often asked by clients why more cannot be done for horses and other large animals when they have broken bones. Technology and orthopaedic advances have revolutionised fracture repairs in other species, including man. Most assume that cost is the deciding factor as to whether an animal is put down or not. There is no doubt that this type of surgery is very expensive, but this is not the reason why most horses with a fracture of a large bone such as a femur, humerus or cannon, have to be euthanased. Indeed, if such a fracture is confirmed the animal is humanely destroyed as soon as possible to stop any further suffering. The sad fact is that despite all the recent advances in surgery, large bone fractures in adult horses and ponies do not heal. In most cases it is not possible to reduce the broken ends of the bone (i.e. put them end to end) and then immobilise them properly, even with stainless-steel pressure plates, to allow healing to take place.

However, there are some cases, especially in young or lightweight ponies where fractures can be reduced and immobilised, and every case should be treated on its own merits and considered properly before any irrevocable decisions are made. It was sad in the case I have just described that a simple minor incident should prove so costly, that nothing more could be done. Had the bone only been split into two or three pieces at the most, then repair might have been possible and it would certainly have been attempted.

Should you ever suspect that your animal has broken a bone – and being suddenly unable to put any weight on a limb is a very diagnostic feature – please get professional help immediately. And please do not move the patient if at all possible until the vet arrives.

CHAPTER TEN

Accidents, First Aid and Self-Medication

Accidents

Most accidents and injuries happen to horses while they are on the move and it is important that a rider or attendant knows what to do.

In the event of an accident, above all stay calm. Your fear and sense of panic will be transmitted to the animal, which will make the situation worse. If on the road, warn oncoming traffic. If it is possible get the horse off the road, but no further if a broken leg is suspected. If the animal is down, put a jacket or something soft under the head to minimise further injury and to stop mud getting in the eye or mouth.

The animal will probably be sweating and trembling. Talk to it, stroke it, reassure and calm it down. Don't attempt to get it up until you are sure it is ready to rise. The horse may just be winded and may want to get up quickly, but if in doubt keep it on the ground until the vet arrives. Cover it over with a blanket or coat or anything that comes to hand that will keep it comfortable.

Before allowing it to stand or before moving the horse make sure the restraint such as the headcollar or halter is adequate for the job. The last thing you want is an injured horse galloping off in a panic.

Wounds

Bleeding wounds are often fairly traumatic, especially if blood is spurting. In these circumstances and if a leg is involved a tourniquet can be applied above the wound. Anything that comes to hand may be used, such as a strip of material, twisted tight with a small bit of wood. However, a tourniquet must not be applied for more than twenty minutes at a time as this might compromise the blood supply to the lower limb. Otherwise, the best way to stop bleeding is by means of a pressure bandage. If blood seeps through, add another layer on top. Any clean material will do in an emergency, but cotton wool/gamgee and elasticated bandages are ideal for the job. If necessary, stop the bleeding by applying firm pressure over the dressing with your hand. Ideally your hand should be clean, but in an emergency don't worry too much.

A wound may be flushed with cold water if the horse is quiet and the wound is grossly contaminated with soil or other debris. If the wound is bleeding heavily do not wash it – it does not stop the flow of blood. Bleeding from the nose can look very serious but usually stops within a few minutes and it does no good to attempt to plug a nostril. It doesn't work and only upsets the horse if you try.

There are four basic types of wound.

• **A contused wound**, which is a term that applies to bruising, can be hosed or bathed with cold water. This reduces the blood-flow to the affected area and reduces swelling and inflammation.

• **A puncture wound** has a very small entrance hole and may bleed heavily to begin with, but a pressure bandage easily controls such haemorrhage.

- **Incised wounds** or cuts are usually clean but depending on the extent and position of the cut will normally require suturing by the vet. This should be done quite quickly, even if bleeding has stopped, while the wound is still fresh. A delay of twenty-four hours or longer may mean the wound will be contaminated and the edges of the cut dried and necrotic, which greatly reduces the chance of the wound healing well.

- **Lacerated wounds** are generally very dirty, fairly superficial and do not bleed very much. This type of wound is typically seen on knees, which have been in contact with a hard surface such as a road. They may be flushed with a cold hose or bathed gently with a saline or antiseptic solution.

Self-medication
The most serious mistake an owner can make in an attempt to save money is to attempt to self-medicate their horse or pony if it goes lame or becomes ill in any way.

Antibiotic sachets or pain-killing preparations such as 'bute' are often hoarded away from previous treatments or borrowed from friends and put into first-aid kits against the day when they might be useful and avoid the necessity and expense of a veterinary visit. Don't do it! I have personally been aware of many cases where this practice is very harmful to the horse and ends up costing the owner more money than it would have done if they had requested professional help from the first instance.

A horse with a foot abscess brewing will initially be only slightly lame and if painkillers or antibiotics are given without knowing the cause of the lameness it could delay the onset of the correct treatment. The effects of the abscess could be much more serious for the patient and the period of lameness and time away from work far more prolonged than need be the case.

I have known one horse which had to be put down due to a broken leg that was initially treated by an owner with some 'bute' she had in her cupboard. The animal had gone lame when it was being exercised. Quite correctly the owner had stopped immediately and box-rested the mare. However, she also gave it some sachets of equipalazone (bute) at the same time, and when the animal became sound very quickly she brought it back into work within a day or two of the initial onset of lameness. It broke its cannon bone when it was next ridden, and although I can't be sure, I suspect the initial lameness may have been a hairline fracture to the bone. The painkillers had masked the symptoms and the owner believed the mare had only suffered some minor bruising. Had she not given the 'bute' the mare would still have been lame and the owner would either have rested the animal longer or sought professional advice. Neither happened, the bone shattered and the horse had to be put down. It was a very expensive, heart-breaking experience.

I know of another animal that had a tendon strain and was put back to work too quickly. It too had been given painkillers that masked symptoms and the tendon ruptured. The animal survived in this case but its athletic career was finished.

Many clients will wish to treat their animals for minor disorders and most of the time little harm will be done, especially if the vet is contacted first for advice, which over the telephone is still given free of charge. Gently bathing a dirty wound with a mild antiseptic solution or hosing a swollen leg before seeking advice will do little harm in the short term providing the condition is obviously improving. If it is not then it is important to know not to persist but seek help.

Just occasionally I come across some self-medication treatments that are very old-fashioned and quite bizarre. The strangest I ever encountered was on Christmas Day about twenty years ago. A client called Barry phoned just after the Queen's speech and asked me to visit.

He had a problem with his horse – it could not pass urine, he said. That was not exactly how he put it but that was what he meant.

I knew Barry quite well and I knew I was usually the last port of call. He would have tried a few home-made remedies before he felt justified in calling out the 'vitnry'.

'What have you given it already?' I asked.

'Not a lot,' he replied. This was not like him at all.

'I don't believe you. You must have given him something.'

'Well, I did stick an onion up his back side,' came the eventual grudging reply. Again, that was not quite what he said but it was the gist of it.

I paused for a moment while trying to think of a suitable answer.

'But why?' was all I could say.

The scorn in his voice was almost palpable. 'Well, everyone knows,' he said, 'that's the best way to make a horse have a piss if it hasn't had one for over a day.'

I could tell he nearly went on to say 'call yourself a vitnry and you don't know that,' but only managed to restrain himself with a huge effort.

Well, as a technique it was all news to me, but for the horse's sake and to get me out of the washing-up, I thought I ought to go along and have a look.

The patient was a nice-looking skewbald colt, which was in some distress. It was sweating a bit, had an elevated pulse rate and was inclined to throw himself on the floor every few minutes in an attempt to roll. It was fairly obvious from the clinical examination that colic was the animal's problem. This was probably the result of constipation, which the onion, being positioned where it was, was doing little to relieve.

The first line of treatment had to be to remove the offending vegetable. As I carried out this delicate operation, the animal got such a fright – well it was the second time that day it had a hand and arm stuck up its bottom – the constipation was relieved in one swift, surprisingly fluid motion. Most of it went over me!

As you can imagine, I was not best pleased with the outcome, even if the horse was instantly feeling better. I turned around to tell Barry exactly what I thought of him and his stupidity only to see him in a heap in the corner, shaking quietly!

Was it an alcoholic convulsion? Was it heck! He had had plenty to drink all right, but he was just having a good laugh at my expense.

After we had both calmed down and order was restored, I collected my equipment. As I was about to leave the stable, the horse passed a large amount of urine and immediately afterwards proceeded to eat its hay from the net as if it had not seen food for at least three days. My lecture to him about never doing that to an animal again somehow lost its point.

The last word was left to Barry who, until his dying day, which was only three years later, was still convinced of the effectiveness of his treatment. 'You just have to give it time to work, vitnry.'

Conclusion

Looking after a horse or pony properly is a huge commitment both in time and money. Spending money properly for regular vaccinations, a well-thought-out worming programme and regular checks on teeth, as well as ensuring proper foot care by a good farrier, is vital for the health and well-being of your animal. It will also save you money in the long term, as it will avoid costly care if your animal becomes ill due to inadequate vaccinations or health care. Many causes of lameness will be avoided by ensuring as far as possible that your horse's feet are properly balanced when being shod or trimmed and that this procedure is carried out at no greater intervals than four to six weeks. A properly balanced diet and adequate exercise are vital for the health of your animal, and time spent in making sure (for example by consulting a vet or nutritionist) that it is eating the correct feed is all-important.

Anyone who has kept a horse or pony will know how it takes over your life. The biggest commitment you can give your horse is time. If you do not have time in a busy lifestyle but still wish to ride occasionally it may be better to use a good riding school or livery yard who will let you hire the horse for a few hours. That way you can leave the health and care to a professional.

Index